LOW SODIUM MEAL RECIPES

The Complete Guide to Breakfast, Lunch, Dinner, and More

(Cook It Yourself With Yummy Low-sodium Main Dish Cookbook!)

Earnestine Morales

Published by Alex Howard

© **Earnestine Morales**

All Rights Reserved

Low Sodium Meal Recipes: The Complete Guide to Breakfast, Lunch, Dinner, and More (Cook It Yourself With Yummy Low-sodium Main Dish Cookbook!)

ISBN 978-1-990169-74-8

Legal & Disclaimer

The information contained in this book is not designed to replace or take the place of any form of medicine or professional medical advice. The information in this book has been provided for educational and entertainment purposes only.

Table of contents

Part 1

Introduction

As mentioned previously, sodium is not all bad for you, in fact you do need sodium in your diet to keep your levels balanced. Sodium is a mineral that does help your body with several functions.

Why is sodium good for you?

Your body needs sodium (or salt) because it regulates your level of electrolytes. When you are sweating, exercising and throughout the day, you will lose some electrolytes that need to be replaced. Your muscles need that certain level of sodium to act properly. Have you ever felt some cramps in your feet or legs? This could very well be caused by too little salt in your diet. Also, your nervous system wants a certain quality of sodium to avoid malfunctions.

Sodium maintains your blood pressure at a normal level if consumed in moderation. Combined with potassium, it acts as regulator of blood pressure and minerals intake (remember we recommend eating bananas when you have body cramps).

According to the dietary guidelines, people should consume approximately 2300 mg of sodium per day. Of course, if your doctor tells to consume less, please follow their recommendations.

Why is sodium bad for you?

Eating foods that contain too much salt can result in your body holding water, causing water retention and that is not a good way to live. A balanced amount of sodium as mentioned before will help your blood pressure to be stable, a higher quantity will elevate the blood pressure to an unhealthy level.

Also, when you blood pressure is too high, there will be some increased risks for many diseases. You would have more chances to develop heart conditions, have a stroke, kidney problems, stomach problems, osteoporosis and even cancer, as well.

Before you have to be on medication for high blood pressure, please monitor your dietary habits carefully. Don't let your sodium consumption cause you some harm. Follow the tips we will share with you in our conclusion and favor some recipes such as the ones included in our cookbook.

Chicken with Bruschetta Topping

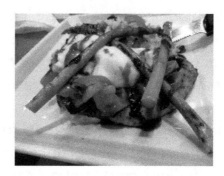

A lot of time to make your chicken tasty, you might tend to add to much salt. Since we want to help you reduce the amount of sodium n your diet, a bruschetta topping seems ideal and here is how you will proceed. I will instruct you how to prepare the dish in the oven, but you could also decide to grill the chicken and it will taste just as fabulous.

Servings: 4

Preparation time: 55 minutes

Ingredients:
- 4 chicken breasts
- 3 medium diced fresh tomatoes
- 2 minced cloves garlic
- 1 small diced red onion
- 2 Tbsp. Fresh chopped parsley

- 1 Tbsp. balsamic vinegar
- 1 Tbsp. olive oil
- Pinch dried cumin
- 1 cup low sodium chicken broth or veggies broth

Method:

1. Preheat the oven to 375 degrees F.
2. Spray with olive oil a large baking dish.
3. In a frying pan, heat the oil and cook the onion with the garlic for 5 minutes. Set aside in a mixing bowl.
4. Add in the bowl, the fresh diced tomatoes and parsley. Also, add the balsamic vinegar and cumin.
5. Place the chicken breasts in the greased dish flat.
6. Add the chicken broth and then add the mixture you prepare on each chicken breasts.
7. Bake in the oven for 45 minutes.
8. Serve with sticky white rice or couscous.

Low Sodium Turkey Pizza

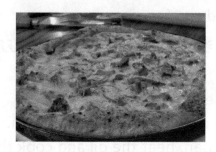

When you think of pizza, you might automatically think of high sodium, but it does not have to be. To avoid a high sodium content, there are a few ways to do so. The cheese and meats you will choose to add as toppings will have a major impact on the overall flavor. Also, the spices and the sauce will have a role to play in this outcome.

Servings: 4

Preparation time: 30-60 minutes

Ingredients:

- 1 cup crumbled goat cheese
- 1 cup chopped smoked turkey
- 1 chopped red onion
- ½ cup marinara sauce
- ½ chopped green bell peppers
- 1 minced Tbsp. garlic
- 1 Tbsp. unsalted butter

Method:

1. Preheat the oven to 400 degrees F.
2. In a pan, heat the unsalted butter and fry for 5 minutes the garlic, the green bell peppers and onion.
3. Add the cooked veggies into the marinara sauce.
4. Spread the marinara sauce on the pizza crust.
5. Add the smoked turkey throughout the pizza.
6. Add also the crumbled goat on the pizza.
7. Bake in the oven for 30-35 minutes and slice away!
8. <u>Perhaps you want to serve with hot sauce or balsamic vinegar.</u>

Delicious Baked Fish Salad

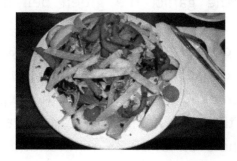

Let's make this beautiful and healthy salad with some baked fish. Adding some deli meats will increase the amount of sodium of your dish, so choosing a baked fish instead is an excellent idea. Although we want to keep it salt free as much as possible, we don't want to compromise the flavor, so let's see how to do so.

Servings: 3-4

Preparation time: 45 minutes

Ingredients:
- 3 medium tilapia filets
- 1 diced avocado
- 4 cups mixed greens
- 1 chopped green onions
- ¼ cup chopped sundried tomatoes

Dressing:
- 1 Tbsp. lemon juice

- 5 Tbs. olive oil
- 1 Tbsp. white balsamic vinegar
- Black pepper
- ½ tsp. garlic powder
- ½ tsp. onion powder
- Pinch smoked paprika

Method:

1. Preheat the oven to 400 degrees F.
2. Season the tilapia filets with pepper and heat some oil in a pan.
3. You will fry the fish for 20 minutes or so or until done.
4. Meanwhile prepare the vinaigrette by missing the following: lemon juice, olive oil, vinegar, black pepper, garlic and onion powder and smoked paprika.
5. Arrange the veggies so when the fish is cooked you can serve the salad right way.
6. Cut the fish in small pieces and divide in 3 or 4 portions.
7. Serve on top of the bed of lettuce with other ingredients.
8. Drizzle some yummy vinaigrette on top and add lemon wedges for presentation if you wish.

Low Sodium Minestrone

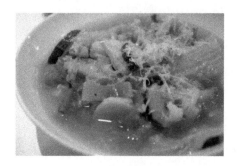

Do not buy canned soups when you are trying to keep your sodium low in your diet. However, it is a great idea to make them form scratch as you can control the exact amount of sodium used with your seasonings. There are many ways to make your soups tasty and low sodium, and you can certainly play with the other spices and herbs until your get your desired flavor.

Servings: 4

Preparation time: 60 minutes

Ingredients:

- 1 cup sliced fresh button mushrooms
- 1 tbsp. minced garlic
- 1 small chopped yellow onion
- 1 cup fresh trimmed green beans
- 1 sliced zucchinis

- 1 can low sodium diced tomatoes
- 5 cups low sodium beef broth
- ¼ cup fresh minced herbs (thyme, oregano, parsley)
- Black pepper

Method:

1. In a large saucepan, heat some oil and cook the garlic, onion, mushrooms and zucchinis for 5 minutes.
2. Add the diced tomatoes and trimmed green beans and cook another 10 minutes.
3. Add the broth with the pepper and all herbs.
4. Bring to boil and cook for another 15 minutes medium-high temperature.
5. Let it simmer until you are ready to serve it.
6. Serve with low sodium grated cheese on top or perhaps a few croutons (Homemade if you prefer).
7. Sometimes I decide to add a cup of cooked shell pasta in the soup, and my kids seems to like it better that way. But that is totally up to you to decide if you want to add rice or pasta.

Potatoes Salad

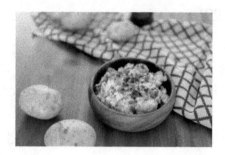

First, let's not boil the potatoes with salt, you will avoid already a good amount of unnecessary salt in this recipe. Then, let's make a nice low sodium sauce to blend well with the cooked potatoes and other ingredients.

Servings: 4

Preparation time: 40 minutes

Ingredients:

- 4 large white potatoes
- 3 Tbsp. minced chives
- 2 cups fresh cauliflower
- 2 minced green onion
- 1 cup sour cream
- Black pepper
- Pinch dried rosemary

- ½ tsp. garlic powder

Method:

1. Peel all the potatoes and cut the cauliflower in florets.
2. Boil water in a large saucepan, cook the potatoes and the cauliflower for about 12-15 minutes.
3. You don't want either of them to become mushy.
4. Remove, drain carefully and set aside to let cool down.
5. In a large bowl, mix the sour cream with the green onions and all seasonings.
6. Add the cooked veggies and mix well.
7. You now have your potatoes salad ready to eat, or store until you are ready to serve it.

Spinach and Ravioli in A Cheese Sauce

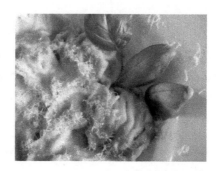

This pasta recipe is fabulous, it involves spinach, raviolis and garlic. It is important to season the dish with other spices than salt, which is essential as the spinach can be pretty bland. Also, the type of cheese you will choose to add will have an impact of the level of sodium in the recipe, so be aware of it.

Servings: 4

Preparation time: 40 minutes

Ingredients:

- 3 cups fresh baby spinach
- 4 servings (3 cups uncooked mushrooms stuffed or pork raviolis)
- 1 Tbsp. minced garlic
- 2 Tbsp. olive oil
- Pinch cayenne pepper

- ¼ cup roasted red peppers

Method:

1. Boil water and cook the raviolis as indicated on the package, normally it takes about 10-12 minutes.
2. Meanwhile, in a large frying pan, heat the olive oil and cook the garlic with e spinach.
3. Add a little of the pasta water to the pan and continue cooking until the pasta is done.
4. Drain the raviolis and add them to the veggies.
5. Stir well and add the roasted pepper as well as the red pepper flakes.
6. Serve with perhaps a little grated Parmesan cheese.

Low Salt Meatloaf

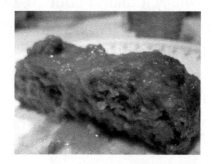

What a healthy way to combine many ingredients together to obtain the most tasteful low sodium meatloaf. First, you should use low fat meat such as ground chicken or turkey and then pay attention to the rest of the seasonings and use salt cautiously.

Servings: 4-6

Preparation time: 60 minutes

Ingredients:

- 1-pound turkey or chicken meat
- ½ cup gluten free breadcrumbs
- ½ cup shredded carrots
- 1 Tbsp. chia seeds
- 1 chopped green onion
- 1 Tbsp... minced garlic
- ½ tsp. dried thyme
- ½ tsp. dried rosemary

- Black pepper
- 1 large egg
- 2 tbsp. whole milk

Topping

- ¼ cup tomato pasta
- 1 Tbsp. molasses
- 1 Tbsp. hot sauce

Method:

1. Preheat the oven to 375 degrees F.
2. Grease a loaf pan and set it aside.
3. In a small pan, heat some butter and cook the garlic and green onions for 5 minutes.
4. In a large mixing bowl, combine the meat, breadcrumbs, milk, chia seeds and all the seasonings.
5. Add the cooked veggies and use your hands to combine the mixture well.
6. Press the meat into the loaf pan.
7. In a separate small bowl, mix the tomato paste, hot sauce and molasses.
8. Add the sauce on top and bake in the oven for 50 minutes.
9. Slice when it cools down and serve with mashed potatoes.

Everyday Seasoned Salmon

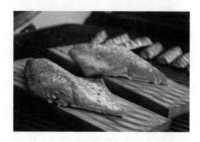

Salmon has a very unique taste on its own so there is no need to add a tone of salt to make it delicious. You should add just enough seasonings to help the taste come out and make it stand out and not kill it with unnecessary salt.

Servings: 4

Preparation time: 45 minutes

Ingredients:

- 4 salmon filets
- 2 tbsp. lemon juice
- 1 Tbsp. minced garlic
- 1 Tbsp. olive oil
- ¼ cup dry white wine
- 1 tbsp. rice vinegar
- 1 tbsp. red pepper flakes
- Pinch dried cumin

- ½ tsp. black pepper

Method:

1. Preheat the oven to 400 degrees F.
2. Grease a rectangle baking dish and set aside.
3. In a pan, heat the olive oil and cook the garlic for 5 minutes.
4. Add the white wine, rice vinegar and the seasonings.
5. This will be poured on the salmon before placing in the oven for about 25 minutes.
6. Serve this delicious salmon with fresh steamed veggies.

Healthy Baked Chicken Wings

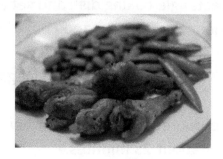

Chicken wings can certainly be included in a low sodium diet, we will need to concentrate a making a great marinade using no or very little salt. You can make them spicy or perhaps with a lot of garlic, which will result in a very tasty and low sodium dish to snack on.

Servings: 4-6

Preparation time: 50-60 minutes

Ingredients:

- 1-pound chicken wings
- ¼ cup low sodium soy sauce
- 2 Tbsp. minced garlic
- 2 minced green onions
- 3 Tbsp. honey
- ¼ cup olive oil or other vegetable oil
- Pinch cayenne pepper

Method:

1. Preheat the oven to 400 degrees F.
2. Spray with non-stick oil a baking sheet and set aside.
3. Clean the chicken wings by patting them down with kitchen towel and season with cayenne pepper.
4. In a large container, combine the soya sauce, olive oil, garlic, green onions, honey.
5. Marinade the chicken wings for at least an hour if you can or even overnight.
6. Bake the wings for 45 minutes or until they are cooked just the way you like them.
7. Serve perhaps with honey mustard dipping sauce.
8. These chicken wings will not be greasy, perhaps s a little sticky, but so tasty, you will not regret it!

Veggies and Cheese Skewers

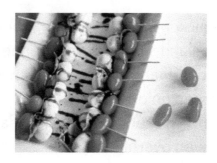

Sometimes finding or preparing some appetizers or snacks that are low in sodium can be a challenge. However, using some low sodium cheeses and veggie it's a great way to ensure you are respecting your restricted diet. I think using the wooden skewers to present them is also fun and original.

Servings: 4-6

Preparation time: 10 minutes

Ingredients:

- 6-12 skewers
- Balsamic vinegar
- 24 cubed Swiss cheese
- 24 cherry or grape tomatoes
- 24-30 baby spinach leaves

Method:

1. Using the Swiss cheese is a good idea, as it is known not to be as salt as other cheese.
2. Use the skewers and start poking through the grape tomatoes, spinach leaves and cheese, alternating each layer.
3. Drizzle the balsamic vinegar on top of the skewers.
4. <u>Place in a serving plate and enjoy!</u>

Fruits and Cottage Cheese Salad

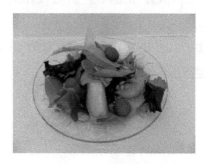

Another way to ensure to keep your sodium intake low is to consume more salads in your regular diet. You really can get away with hardly any salt if you are careful about the salad dressing you will use and the other toppings, such as croutons or nuts.

Servings: 4

Preparation time: 15 minutes

Ingredients:

- 4-5 cups mixed kale and spinach or other mixed greens of your choice
- 2 cups sliced strawberries
- 1/2 cup unsalted walnuts
- 1 cup cottage cheese or ricotta cheese
- Oil and vinegar dressing
- Black pepper

Method:

1. On individual plates or bowls, place the mixed greens, sliced strawberries and a generous portion of low salt cheese.
2. Add some walnuts on top.
3. In a bowl, mix the oil, vinegar and black pepper.
4. Drizzle the dressing on top of the salad and enjoy as a light lunch any day.
5. You could also add some grilled chicken or tuna to the dish if you want to have a protein in your meal.
6. Also, to add additional proteins, you can sprinkle some chia seeds in your dressing prior to pouring it on your salad.

Perfectly Sautéed Ground Beef in Lettuce Wraps

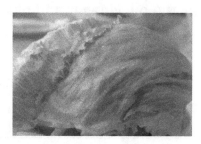

Let's make some very healthy lettuce wraps, and let's make them low sodium please. One way to make sure it stays low in sodium is to avoid adding certain cheeses in the preparation and that is exactly what we are going to do here.

Servings: 4

Preparation time: 35-40 minutes

Ingredients:

- 4-8 large lettuce leaves (Romaine is great for this)
- ½ ground beef meat
- 1 Tbsp. hot sauce
- 2 tbsp. minced parsley
- Black pepper
- 1 shredded zucchinis

- 1 Tbsp. olive oil

Method:

1. Grate or shred the zucchinis finely.
2. In a pan, heat the olive oil and start cooking the meat and zucchinis together.
3. Add the hot sauce, parsley and black pepper after 10 minutes or so.
4. Stir often so the meat stays crumbly.
5. When the meat is cooked, display the lettuce leaves in the serving plates.
6. Add a generous portion of the meat and zucchinis mixture into the lettuce leaves and enjoy!
7. Add more hot sauce if needed.

Apples and Nuts Cup

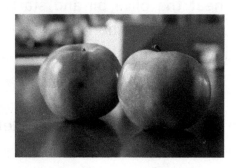

You might think that desserts do not need to use salt at all, but honestly it is not always the case. However, this recipe is lets you enjoy the sweet flavors without asking you to add salt, so perfect dessert for this cookbook. Shall we start?

Servings: 4

Preparation time: 35-40 minutes

Ingredients:

- 4 cups favorite sliced red apples (Gala works well)
- 4 Tbsp. cashew butter (unsalted)
- 2 Tbsp. agave syrup
- ¼ cup water
- Pinch cinnamon
- 1 cup chopped pecans

Method:

1. In a medium saucepan, place the apples, water, cinnamon and agave syrup. Bring to boil.
2. Continue cooking for 20 minutes on medium high temperature, until apples are soft. Stir a few times. Let the apples cool down before you assemble.
3. Take 4 desserts cups and place a generous portion of the apples in the bottom.
4. Spread a tablespoon of cashew butter on top and add the pecans as final topping.
5. <u>Enjoy with some wiped cream if you like or even vanilla ice cream.</u>

Low Sodium Quesadillas

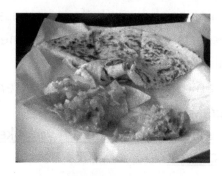

Making some wonderful Mexican simple dishes is totally possible without using too much salt. You should focus on using some fresh veggies and herbs, and avoid adding cheese, or look to add low sodium cheese instead or regular. Also, be careful when you season the meat and vegetables used.

Servings: 4

Preparation time: 30 minutes

Ingredients:

- ¼ pound chicken strips
- 1 sliced red bell pepper
- 1 sliced small sweet onion
- 1 Tbsp. olive oil
- 1 tbsp. chili powder
- ½ tsp. black pepper

- ½ cup shredded Monterey Jack cheese
- 4 medium size tortilla breads
- <u>Sour cream and diced fresh tomatoes as condiments as you wish</u>

Method:

1. Season the chicken strips with chili powder.
2. Heat oil in the large frying pan and start cooking the chicken strips.
3. Add the red bell pepper, onions and continue cooking for another 10-12 minutes.
4. Season the veggies with black pepper and chili powder.
5. When ready to assemble, lay a tortilla bread, add your desired condiments, including the cheese and a generous portion of chicken and veggies.
6. <u>Heat a few more drops of oil and fold the tortilla bread in half to start grilling in the pan. Flip after 5 minutes or until you are satisfied.</u>

Asian Shrimp and Fruits Skewers

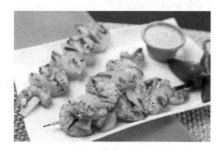

These skewers are so delightful and kind of refreshing, I must say. My personal favorite is the fresh diced pineapple with shrimp, cooked on the grill. However, it could be any of your favorite fruits, such as oranges, mangoes or strawberries. Just beware of the size of the fruits when you grill them, so they stay on the skewers well during the cooking session.

Servings: 4-6

Preparation time: 30-60 minutes

Ingredients:

- ½ pound shrimp (deveined and peeled)
- 2 tbsp. lime juice
- 1 tbsp. lime zest
- 2 Tbsp. minced garlic
- Pinch turmeric
- 3 tbsp. olive oil

- ½ tsp. red pepper flakes
- ½ diced fresh pineapple or about1 cup

Method:

1. Turn on the grill on medium high temperature.
2. Meanwhile, in a mixing bowl, combine the lime juice, lime zest, minced garlic, red pepper flakes and turmeric.
3. Marinade the shrimp for at least an hour if you can.
4. Assemble the shrimp and pineapple on the skewers, alternating each layer.
5. Grill for about 7-8 minutes on each side.
6. Serve on a bed of rice with lime wedges on the side.

Low Salt Brownies

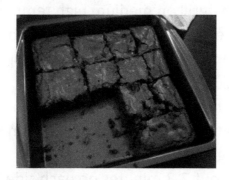

Salt in desserts can bring out the sweetness of it, but if you use the right additional ingredients, no need to worry about added salt. Also, you must avoid using salty nuts of course, if you decide to use nuts. It is important to understand all the source where salt is sometimes hidden.

Servings: 8-12

Preparation time: 50 minutes

Ingredients:

- 2 tbsp. unsalted butter
- ¼ cup apple sauce
- 2 medium eggs
- ¾ cup brown sugar
- 4 Tbsp. unsweetened cocoa
- ¼ cup bitter sweet chocolate chips

- ½ cup all-purpose flour
- 1 tsp. vanilla extract
- ½ tsp. baking soda
- ½ tsp. baking powder

Method:

1. Preheat the oven to 350 degrees F.
2. Grease a square baking pan and set aside.
3. In a large mixing bowl, combine all dry ingredients: cocoa, brown sugar, flour, baking powder and baking soda.
4. In a second bowl, mix the eggs, vanilla, apple sauce and butter.
5. Add the wet ingredients to the dry ones and combine with a wooden spoon.
6. Finally, add the chocolate chips to the mixture and pour into the baking dish.
7. Bake for about 40 minutes.
8. Let the brownies cool down and cut into squares.

Spinach Apples and Lemon Dressing

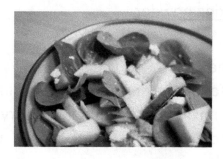

This yummy salad does not need salt to taste good. It however needs that very unique salad dressing we will help you perfect. You can use that dressing on other of your favorite salads. You can also use kale or other mixed greens and pears instead of apples, and this will still be a perfectly healthy and low sodium option.

Servings: 4-6

Preparation time: 30-60 minutes

Ingredients:

- 4 cups baby spinach leaves
- 2 large Granny Smith sliced apples
- 1 sliced small English cucumber (seedless)
- 1 diced pitted avocado
- 5-6 sliced radishes
- 5 Tbsp. avocado oil

- 2 Tbsp. sesame seeds
- 2 Tbsp. lemon juice
- 1Tbps. minced garlic
- 1 Tbsp. minced ginger
- ½ tsp. Dijon mustard
- Black pepper
- Few mint leaves

Method:

1. Prepare the dressing first to make sure all the flavors have time to mix well together.
2. So, in a mixing bowl, mix the oil, sesame seeds, lemon juice, garlic, ginger, mustard, mint leaves and black pepper.
3. Get 4 plates out and divide the spinach equally among the plates.
4. Add some sliced apple and cucumber, diced avocado and radishes as you please.
5. Top if off with the delicious vinaigrette you created.
6. If you want to make it a meal, add some cooked turkey or chicken.

Amazing Chicken, Noodles and Veggies Soup

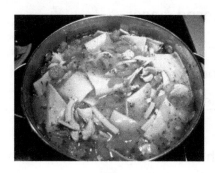

When you think of canned soups, you think high sodium automatically. That's why it is always better to make your soups homemade as much as possible. Chicken noodles soups can be very yummy without all that added salt, use fresh and dried herbs instead and other flavorful ingredients which we will suggest below.

Servings: 4-6

Preparation time: 60 minutes

Ingredients:

- 6 cups low fat chicken
- 1 large sliced carrot
- 1 Tbsp. minced garlic
- ½ chopped yellow onion
- 1 large sliced white or yellow peeled potato

- 1 cup uncooked macaroni noodles
- 1 Tbsp. fresh minced thyme
- 1 Tbsp. minced fresh parsley
- Black pepper
- 1 cup shredded cooked chicken
- 1 Tbsp. unsalted butter

Method:

1. In a large saucepan, heat the butter, cook the onion and garlic until soft.
2. In a separate saucepan, boil water and cook the potato and carrot for 15 minutes.
3. Add the cooked sliced potatoes and carrots to the first saucepan.
4. Also add the chicken broth, bring to boil and add the noodles.
5. Add finally all the herbs and spices.
6. Continue cooking for another 30 minutes or so. Serve with unsalted cracker or pita bread.

Cauliflower Patties

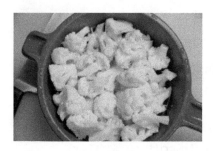

Because cauliflower is good for you, but not everyone's favorite, we thought of sharing this simple and different recipe which might make it more enjoyable. The fact that we make patties with the veggie makes it very unique, but to avoid adding tone of salt, we will also serve it with some fresh made bruschetta on top. See below for further instruction.

Servings: 4-6

Preparation time: 30-60 minutes

Ingredients:
- 4 cups cooked cauliflower
- 1 small can rinsed and drained chickpeas
- 2 large eggs
- ¼ cup gluten free breadcrumbs
- ½ tsp. smoked paprika
- ½ tsp. Ground cumin

- ½ tsp. onion powder
- ½ tsp. garlic powder
- Frying oil (coconut oil or other vegetable oil)

Topping

- 1 diced pitted avocado
- 1 cup diced fresh tomatoes
- 1 Tbsp. minced garlic
- 1 Tbsp. olive oil
- Pinch cumin
- Black pepper
- 1 Tbsp. lime juice

Method:

1. In a food processor, add the cooked cauliflower and chickpeas. Blend, until you are left with what looks like a paste almost.
2. Place this mixture in a bowl and add the breadcrumbs, the eggs and all spices.
3. Heat the frying oil in the pan.
4. Form with your hands the patties and fry them for 7-8 minutes on each side. Once they are done, lay them on paper towels to absorb the excess oil.
5. Meanwhile, prepare the topping.
6. Dice the avocados and the tomatoes, place them in a bowl.
7. Add in the bowl the lime juice, olive oil, cumin and pepper.

8. Mix well and place on top of each petty when serving.

9. <u>This makes a great appetizer or a side dish, as you wish.</u>

Low Salt Fried Rice

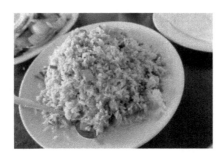

When you order fried rice at the Chinese restaurant, you will get a meal that is very high in sodium. We want to avoid this, so why don't you make it yourself at home instead. We will use low sodium ingredients and you will realize how tasty it can be with all these high sodium sauce added.

Servings: 4

Preparation time: 40 minutes

Ingredients:

- 4 cups cooked brown rice
- 1 cup sweet peas
- 1 Tbsp. minced garlic
- 3 chopped green onions
- 2 Tbsp. sesame oil
- 2 tbsp. sesame seeds

- 1 chopped red bell pepper
- 2 Tbsp. soy sauce (reduce sodium)
- Pinch cayenne pepper
- 2 cups diced cooked pork

Method:

1. I love making fried rice any day of the week.
2. If you don't have left over rice, use vegetables broth to cook your rice, low sodium, of course, to add some additional flavor to the dish.
3. In a large pan, heat the sesame oil and cook the sesame seeds and garlic together for 5 minutes.
4. Add the red bell pepper and green onions and cook an additional 10 minutes.
5. Then, add the cooked rice, soy sauce and pork. Sir all the ingredients together well.
6. Sprinkle some cayenne pepper and continue cooking for another 10-15 minutes on low temperature.
7. Serve hot in bowls or plates, your choice.

Chicken Curry

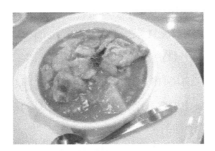

Salt is a key ingredient to many dishes. However, when you decide to cook curried chicken, you can still do it while minimizing the sodium content. Curry is a very unique spice, it can be overwhelming if you use too much, so pay attention and taste and adjust instead of adding too much to begin with.

Servings: 4

Preparation time: 45 minutes

Ingredients:

- 1 can coconut milk
- 1 small chopped yellow onion
- 1 chopped red bell pepper
- 2 tbsp. red curry paste
- Pinch dried ginger
- Black pepper
- ½ pound chicken tenders
- 2 Tbsp. olive oil

- ¼ cup sliced black olives
- 1 small can drained bamboo shoots

Method:

1. In a large pan, heat the olive oil.
2. Season the chicken tenders with black pepper.
3. Start sautéing the chicken in the pan with the bell pepper and onions for about 20 minutes.
4. In a small saucepan, mix the coconut milk with the curry paste and the dried ginger.
5. Stir for 5-10 minutes while bringing to boil and then reduce the heat to low temperature.
6. Add the sauce the chicken and add the black olives and bamboo shoots.
7. Serve the chicken with the sauce, veggies and all on a bed of rice or couscous or even quinoa.

Berries and Yogurt

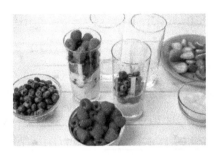

It's enjoyable to make low sodium desserts any chance we get. We ingest enough sodium as it is when we prepare other dishes and main courses. Desserts do not need to be salty! Let's make them sweet, but also as healthy as possible, using some natural sources of glucose. Here is one way below.

Servings: 3-4

Preparation time: 15 minutes

Ingredients:

- 1 medium banana
- 1 cup fresh blueberries
- 1 Tbsp. flaxseeds
- 1 cup Ricotta cheese
- 1 cup plain Greek yogurt
- Pinch cinnamon
- Pinch nutmeg

Method:

1. You can use a high sped blender or a food processor for this recipe.
2. Combine all the ingredients in your chosen device.
3. Activate and then pour the mixture into 3-4 bowls.
4. You can also leave it in a storage container and keep it in the fridge and get a portion as you need or want one during the week.
5. Sprinkle extra flaxseeds or granola on top of the yogurt when you are serving if you like.
6. <u>You can also keep a few fresh fruits blueberries) and decorate when serving on top.</u>

Seared Tuna

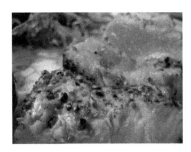

Seared tuna is a very popular item on the menus these days, but why not make it at home, so you can enjoy it at lower cost. You must absolutely have confidence in your point of purchase, make sure you do buy some very fresh tuna. Then, equip yourself with a great knife and some fresh vegetables as sides. You will find the low sodium teriyaki sauce usually in specialized store, such as Asian markets. If not, ask your grocery store manager to order some for you.

Servings: 4-6

Preparation time: 30-60 minutes

Ingredients:

- 3 fresh tuna filets
- 3 Tbsp. teriyaki sauce, low sodium
- 1 Tbsp. minced garlic
- 2 Tbsp. lemon juice

- 1 Tbsp. smoked paprika
- 2 cups cooked quinoa
- Served with minced ginger
- Some wasabi paste

Method:

1. I strongly suggest marinating the fresh tuna overnight. If you can't a few hours will do.
2. In a bowl, mix the teriyaki sauce, garlic, lemon juice, and smoke paprika.
3. Place the fresh cut tuna fish in a storage container with a top. You don't want to leave it open, you want to avoid contamination as you will not cook the tuna fully.
4. Once you are ready to sear the tuna, make sure all the other sides are ready.
5. Cook the quinoa, slice the fresh ginger and plate it.
6. Heat a few drops of olive oil in the pan and sear the tuna, meaning simply cook it for 1 minute or so on each side.
7. Plate the seared tuna on a bed of quinoa with sliced ginger and wasabi pasta on the side, it will be a beautiful dish to serve your guests or you husband on a Saturday night
8. Pour yourself a glass of dry white wine.

Beans and Pasta Salad

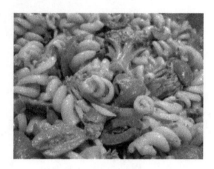

This pasta salad will be so nutritive and so colorful at the same time. The beans you will be adding to the salad will be an excellent source of protein. Then, you will add some awesome herbs, vegetables and yes, a few fruits also.

Servings: 4-6

Preparation time: 40 minutes

Ingredients:
- 1 cup drained white kidney beans
- 1 cup drained red kidney beans
- ½ cup minced red onion
- 1 cup diced peaches (fresh is always better, but you can use the ones in can, low sugar, low sodium)
- 1 box cooked penne pasta
- 1 Tbsp. black pepper

- 1 tsp. dried coriander
- 1 box uncooked fusilli pasta
- 4 cups vegetables broth
- 1 cup plain Greek yogurt
- ½ tsp. Dijon mustard

Method:

1. Boil the vegetables broth in a pot and cook the pasta as you normally would or as indicated on the box.
2. Once the pasta is cooked, drain well and set aside in a large mixing bowl.
3. In another bowl, mix the yogurt, mustard, coriander, pepper.
4. Add the yogurt sauce to the pasta and mix.
5. Add next the rest of the ingredients to the pasta salad; drained beans, diced peaches, diced red onion.
6. Combine once more and serve or refrigerate until ready to serve.

Brussel Sprouts in Sauce

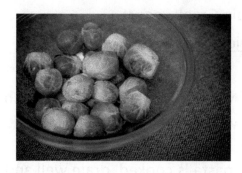

Brussel sprouts are not only very rich is vitamins and minerals, but also good for you. You should definitely add them in your low sodium diet. I will say that I have been guilty in the past for adding way too much salt when serving sprouts, but I am learning to serve them differently now.

Servings: 4-6

Preparation time: 45 minutes

Ingredients:

- 4 cups fresh Brussel sprouts
- 6 cooked bacon slices (low sodium turkey bacon)
- 2 tbsp. honey
- 1 cup apple juice
- 1 Tbsp. minced garlic
- ½ tbsp. red pepper flakes

Method:

1. You will want to boil some water in a large pot and cook the Brussel sprouts for about 20 minutes.
2. They should not get mushy, but they should soften a lot.
3. In a large pan, meanwhile, cook the bacon and set aside when it is cooked. Keep the bacon grease in the pan.
4. Add the apple juice, garlic and honey to the bacon grease and cook the garlic for 5 minutes.
5. Add the Brussel sprouts and cook another 10 minutes on medium heat.
6. Finally, sprinkle the bacon crumbs and stir once more before serving.

Low Sodium Breakfast Recipes

Chocolate Hazelnut Crepes with Fruits

Ingredients

Chocolate hazelnut spread (1 cup)

Crepes (4 in number)

4 sliced bananas

1 can whipped cream (pressurized)

Directions

Evenly spread out the hazelnut flavored spread on each crepe. Place a sliced banana at the center of the crepe and then roll it up. Place this into a warm pan over medium heat and then let the stay warm for two minutes. Move them to a plate and top up with the whipped cream.

French Toast with Peaches & Mascarpone

Ingredients

8 peaches (fresh)

1/2 cup white sugar

4 bolillo rolls (Mexican)

1 cup cheese (mascarpone)

6 tbsp sugar (confectioners')

1 zested lemon

4 pinches of nutmeg (grounded)

1/2 tsp cinnamon (grounded)

6 big eggs

3/4 cup fresh milk

Vanilla extract (1/2 tsp)

Butter (2 tsp)

Vegetable oil (2 tsp)

Directions

Remove the skin from the peaches and pit them. Slice them into a saucepan and stir in nutmeg, sugar and cinnamon and cook this over a medium heat until you can see bubbles. Stir the mixture as it cooks and continue to do this until the sauce runs like a syrup. This will take a time of 10 minutes and when it Is ready take the pan away from the heat.

Cut the bolillo rolls at the end and then slice them into thick slices. Place each slice on a flat surface and then cut a pocket onto each size leaving three sides of the roll intact. Place them aside.

Add the confectioners' sugar and mascarpone, lemon zest and sugar and place this mixture into a plastic bag. Snip off one corner of the bag and fill it with as much filling. Fill pocket into slice of bread without overflowing it.

In a bowl, whisk the vanilla, eggs and milk and then melt oil over medium heat in a different pan. Dip each stuffed bread piece into the batter and put into the pan and then cook till all sides are brown. Serve while they peach sauce is still warm.

Almond Crunch Granola

Ingredients

1 cup slivered toasted almonds

1 cup coconut (flaked)

1/2 cup of honey

2 1/2 cups of rolled oats

3/4 tsp of cinnamon

1/4 cup vegetable or almond

Direction

Mix the coconut, oats, and cinnamon with toasted almonds. Blend honey and oil and drizzle this over the oats and almonds mixture. Toss them together and then cook this in an oven heated to 350 degrees F for a period of thirty minutes. Stir often as it cooks and when time has elapsed, get it out of the oven and loosen it using a spatula then leave it to cool down.

Classic Hash Browns

Ingredients

2 peeled russet potatoes

3 tbsp butter (clarified)

Grounded black pepper

Table salt

A pinch of cayenne pepper

A pinch of paprika

Directions

Shred the russet potatoes into a bowl that contains cold water and then stir the water until the water is cloudy in appearance. Drain the potatoes and run cold water through them again to remove any starch that remained on them. Drain the water off of the potatoes and pat them dry on a paper towel.

In a non stick pan heat the butter over medium heat and then sprinkle in the shredded potatoes. Season them with all the peppers, salt and paprika.

Cook them until there is a layer of brown crust underneath the pan. This will take a time of five minutes. Cook until all the potatoes have become brown.

French Toast & Spiced Pears

Ingredients

Honey (3 tbsp)

Lemon juice (1 tbsp)

1/4 tsp cinnamon (grounded)

1/4 tsp ginger (grounded)

2 large ripe cored pears (sliced)

2 big eggs

Honey (1 tbsp)

1/4 tsp cinnamon (grounded)

1/4 tsp ginger (grounded)

1/3 cup fresh milk

4 slices of bread

1/4 cup of toasted almonds (sliced)

Directions

Set the oven to 175 degrees C or 350 degrees F and let it preheat. As the oven heats, grease the baking tin that will be used to prepare the dish.

Make a mixture put of mixing ¼ tsp of ginger and the same amount of cinnamon mixed with lemon juice into a bowl. Pour this mixture into the already prepared baking dish then arrange the pears at the bottom.

In another bowl, add ¼ tsp of ginger and ¼ tsp of cinnamon and beat eggs into the same bowl. Dip each slice of bread into the egg mixture and the place then on top of the arranged pears.

Bake this in the oven which was preheated until the bread turns brown and has set. This takes a time of twenty minutes.

Slice the bread into square shapes and then lift it off the baking dish using a spatula. Now the side with the pears will be facing upwards. Sprinkle this side with almonds and drizzle the syrup that remains on the baking dish onto the top.

Banana Bran Muffins

Ingredients

2 egg whites

1 tsp of grounded cinnamon

1/8 tsp grounded nutmeg

2 tbsp olive oil (light)

Mashed banana (1 cup)

Baking powder (3 tbsp)

Oat bran (2 cups)

Skim milk (1/2 a cup)

Directions

Set the oven to 220 °C or 425 °F and let it preheat. Meanwhile lightly spray muffin cups that you will use using cooking spray.

Mix all the dry ingredients into one bowl.

Mix the egg whites, mashed banana and oil in another bowl and combine them well until they are blended together.

Pour out this wet mixture into the previously prepared dry ingredients. Mix them well.

When mixed, pour the combined mixture into the prepared muffin tins.

Bake them till they change color to golden brown. This takes a time of not more than 20 minutes.

Turkey Sausage Patties

Ingredients

½ tsp fresh basil leaves

Coriander (1 tsp)

Cumin (1/2 tsp)

Garlic powder (1/2 tsp)

½ tsp oregano leaves

Paprika (1 tsp)

Black pepper (1/4 tsp)

Cayenne pepper (1/2 tsp)

1 pound of grounded turkey

½ a cup the broth of chicken

Directions

Mix together all the spices and turkey in a bowl and then ensure that you combine them well.

Pour in the broth from the chicken and let this sit together for a time of not more than 20 minutes.

Mould the turkey into sizeable patties with a thickness of 3/4".

Go ahead and cook the patties on a non stick pan over medium heat for a time of eight minutes for every side until they are well cooked.

Watermelon Mania

Ingredients

Watermelon (110 grams)

Cubes of iced water (15 in number)

Directions

Remove the seeds from the watermelon and place it and the ice cubes into a blender.

To spruce it up, add some redbull or diet soda.

Blend all these together to a fine consistency.

Drink is ready to be served.

Crock Pot Oatmeal

Ingredients

Cinnamon (1 tsp)

2 ½ cups oatmeal

12 oz chopped apple

Raisins (1/2 a cup)

6 cups of plain water

Directions

Put all the ingredients into a crock pot and the mix them well and cook them over night over a very low heat.

Add sweetener to give it a taste.

Breakfast Sausage

Ingredients

Lean fresh ground pork (8 ounces), preferably 80% lean

Chicken/Vegetable stock (2 tbsp)

Red pepper flakes (1/2 tsp)

Dried Thyme (1/2 tsp)

Dried Sage (1/4 tsp)

Black pepper (1/2 tsp)

Directions

Mix all the ingredients in a bowl thoroughly. Take the mixture and divide equally into 8 portions (about 1 tsp each portion) and roll them balls on a sheet of waxed paper (folded in half). Place all the balls on one side of the waxed paper and fold over the other side. Press the balls into patties.

Cook on a skillet sprayed with cooking spray, over medium-high heat for about 10 minutes, turning halfway. Cook until the internal temperature reaches 160 degrees F.

Conclusion

Few tips to avoid using too much sodium in the kitchen

1. Simply do not put the salt shaker on the table, then you avoid temptation of adding salt to your dishes.
2. Use fresh, natural meats, and avoid deli meats or processed meats
3. Instead of adding salt to your dish, try adding herbs or garlic.
4. Adding some lemon juice or unsalted bouillon can also add a lot of flavors to your meals without the high content of sodium.
5. Use some non-salted or low salted canned foods, or avoid them all together (soups, vegetables, beans).
6. Avoid salted nuts, always choose the unsalted ones.
7. Always read the food labels carefully, sodium should not be listed on top of the list.
8. Avoid eating out when you can or choose low sodium items.
9. Reduce your overall potion sizes, less food, less sodium, it is as simple as that.
10. Make sure you taste your food before adding any salt, most of the time, we do add sodium by habit and not because it needs extra flavoring!
11. Avoid of course all processed and extra salty foods such as pretzels, chips, crackers or look for low sodium options.

We surely hope you enjoyed learning about sodium and cooking with less sodium. We value your well-being and your happiness. So, our purpose was to provide you some excellent recipes to keep you super healthy. Enjoy!

Part 2

Main Dishes

Home Fries | Low Sodium Version

Potatoes become very bad for health when deep-fried in oil. But still fries are a main component of all junk food meals. In order to enjoy fries without the added disadvantages of deep fried things, here is a recipe that will let you enjoy fries without the guilt. This recipe can be doubled or tripled but must be consumed within the day.

Preparation Time: 10 minutes

Cooking Time: 20 minutes

Serving: Single cup serving for 2 people

Sodium per Serving: 148mg

Ingredients

☐ Red Yukon Gold Potatoes 8 ounces (Diced)

☐ Spray Oil

☐ Onion 1 small (Diced)

☐ Salt 1/8 tsp

☐ Fresh Ground Black Pepper

Directions

Take a glass bowl and arrange the diced potatoes in it. Microwave the potatoes for one minute on high and then stir them through and leave them aside.

Warm up a large non-stick skillet over medium-high heat and spray with oil. Cook the diced onions in it by stirring and tossing till the onions are of a light brown color. During this process, microwave the potatoes on high for one minute again. Stir them and let them rest for a minute and then repeat the process again.

After the onions are done, throw in the microwaved potatoes and seasonings. Spray a bit of oil again and cook the potatoes till they are light brown in color. Keep tossing to prevent the home fries from getting stuck to the bottom of the pan.

Asian Lettuce Wraps | Low Sodium Version

Asian style cooking has its distinct aroma and presentation. Making stuffed parcels of lettuce is not just catchy but also fun to eat. This recipe can be multiplied as many times as you want to and you can refrigerate whatever is left of the stuffing for nearly three days.

Preparation Time: 15 minutes

Cooking Time: 30 minutes

Serving: Single cup serving for 1 person

Sodium per Serving: 246 mg

Ingredients

- ☐ Water 2 cup
- ☐ Brown Rice 1/3 cup
- ☐ Sesame Oil 2 tsp
- ☐ Red Onion (Diced) 1 medium
- ☐ Carrot (Diced) 1 large
- ☐ Ribs Celery (Diced) 2 large
- ☐ Fresh Ginger (Minced) 2 Tbsp
- ☐ Low Sodium Chicken or Vegetable Broth ½ cup
- ☐ Fresh Ground Black Pepper
- ☐ Red Pepper Flakes 1/8 tsp
- ☐ Hoisin Sauce 2 Tbsp

- ☐ Boneless Skinless Chicken Thighs (Diced)   8 ounces
- ☐ Water 1 cup
- ☐ Red Bell Pepper (Diced)   ¼ medium
- ☐ Cilantro Leaves ¼ cup
- ☐ Leaves Iceberg Lettuce (Rinsed and Patted dry)   8 medium

Directions

In order to cook the rice, take a medium sized pot and boil the water in it. Once it reaches boiling point, add the rice to it and stir. Reduce the heat to moderate and allow the rice to simmer for nearly fifteen minutes. Put a lid on the pot but cover it only partially and do not stir. Don't let all the liquid dry out, so when only a little liquid is left, remove the pot from heat and over it completely. Leave it to stand for a while.

While the rice is simmering, take a large sauté pan and warm up the sesame oil in it. Drop the onions in it and stir fry till the onions are caramelized. Do not let the onions get dark brown and keep the heat moderately high.

Once the onions are done, lower the heat and add the ginger, celery and carrots. Cook for a couple of minutes and add the diced chicken. Keep on stirring to evenly cook the vegetables and chicken. After a couple of minutes add the stock and the sauces. Stir in the water and reduce the heat even more,

Place a lid halfway over the pan and let the mixture cook for ten to fifteen minutes. The water should be nearly dried up. Then add the red pepper flakes to it and stir in the cooked rice. Stir the mixture for one more minute and remove from heat.

To serve, place the mixture in a large bowl and four lettuce leaves per person. Then place a scoop of the mixture in the middle of lettuce leaf and drop a tablespoon of cilantro onto the scoop and roll up the leaf.

Asian Peanut Chicken with Noodles

Peanuts have a creamy toasty flavor that works well with chicken. This recipe is a versatile one because the leftovers can be utilized in different salads. You can multiply the recipe as many times as you want.

Preparation Time: 10 minutes

Cooking Time: 20 minutes

Serving: 2 ounce pasta with 3 ounces chicken and sauce serving for 2 people

Sodium per Serving: 257 mg

Ingredients

☐ Water   3 quarts

☐ Smooth Peanut Butter 3 Tbsp

☐ Fresh Cilantro Leaves ¼ cup

☐ Lime (Juiced) ½

☐ Low-Sodium soy sauce 2 tsp

☐ Low Sodium Chicken or Vegetable Broth2 Tbps

☐   Boneless Skinless Chicken Breast (Sliced into Strips) 6 ounces

☐ Frozen Edamame (Soybeans)   ½ cup

☐ Whole Wheat or Gluten-free Spaghetti4 ounces

☐ Carrot (Shredded) 1 small

☐ Red Onion (Slivered; to taste)

☐ Dry Roasted Unsalted Peanuts   2 Tbsp

First of all preheat the oven to a moderate heat of 200°. You have to puree the peanut butter, lime juice, stock, soy sauce, cilantro and red pepper flakes. You could use a food processor or blender for this purpose. But the end result should be a smooth paste.

Boil three quarts of the water in a large saucepan on a high flame. Lower the flame when the water reaches boiling point and let it simmer. Blanch the chicken strips in it for five minutes and then remove with the help of tongs. Do not drain the water and place the chicken in the oven to cook some more.

Once the chicken is in the oven, increase the heat under the water and once it is back to boiling point, add the pasta to it. Cook the pasta for around ten minutes before adding the edamame. Then cook further for a minute. Take out ½ cup of the pasta water and reserve it. Drain the pasta and edamame and return to the now empty saucepan. Keep the heat moderate and add the peanut sauce, baked chicken, onions and shredded carrots. Keep tossing the mixture and cook for half a minute more before removing from heat

If the sauce gets too thick then dilute it bit by bit, with the reserve pasta water. Decorate it with peanuts and serve it hot.

Asian Turkey Burgers | Low Sodium Version

Using turkey in a burger is a good way to experiment with the meat portion of a burger. You can creative with how you serve this burger because of its tangy taste. The burger should be consumed within the day because it can't be stored well and you can multiply it as many times as you want.

Preparation Time: 10 minutes

Cooking Time: 20 minutes

Serving: 1 quarter pound hamburger serving for 2 people

Sodium per Serving: 480 mg

Ingredients

- ☐ Garlic (Minced) 1 clove
- ☐ Shallot (Minced) 1 small
- ☐ Ginger (Peeled and Minced)1 Tbsp
- ☐ Lime Juice ¼ cup
- ☐ Cayenne Pepper 1/8 tsp
- ☐ Fresh Ground Black Pepper (To taste)
- ☐ Ground Turkey (Breast is Better) 8 ounces
- ☐ Olive Oil 2 tsp
- ☐ Hoisin Sauce 1 Tbsp
- ☐ Brown Sugar 1 tsp

- ☐ Low-Sodium Soy Sauce   1 tsp
- ☐ Red Pepper Flakes   1/8 tsp
- ☐ Spray Olive Oil
- ☐ Whole Wheat or Gluten-free Hamburger buns   2

Directions

You can either grill the patties or bake them. So preheat the grill or preheat the oven to 400°F.

Toss together the ground turkey, lime juice, cayenne pepper, ginger, garlic and shallot. When they are thoroughly mixed, shape the mixture into two hamburger patties.

In a small bowl, mix the hoisin sauce, brown sugar, olive oil, red pepper flakes and soy sauce. This is the basting sauce.

Now place a grill pan in the oven while it preheats and once it is hot, spray it lightly with oil. If you are using the grill then allow it to heat up and then spray oil over it. Place the burgers on the grill and then drip some of the basting sauce over the patties.

Cook one side for five minutes and then flip over. Baste again and cook for three minutes. Repeat the process till the basting sauce is finished and then cook around five more minutes. Serve the burgers on toasted buns.

Barbeque Chicken

This is a very easy recipe to make and the leftovers can be utilized in a multitude of ways. You can serve it with different things to add to the delicious flavor of this chicken, which also works well on its own. This recipe can be multiplied as many times as desired.

Preparation Time: 5 minutes

Cooking Time: 25 minutes

Serving: 1 chicken piece and ¼ cup sauce serving for 8 people

Sodium per Serving: 126 mg

Ingredients

- ☐ Low-Sodium Ketchup   1 cup
- ☐ Apricot Jelly ¼ cup
- ☐ Dark Brown Sugar   ¼ cup
- ☐ Cider Vinegar ½ cup
- ☐ Worcestershire Sauce   1 Tbsp
- ☐ Water 2 tsp
- ☐ Hot Sauce 1/8 tsp
- ☐ Garlic Powder 1/8 tsp
- ☐ Dry Mustard ½ tsp
- ☐ Chili Powder 1 tsp

- ☐ Paprika 1 tsp
- ☐ Ground Black Pepper   1 tsp
- ☐ Piece per Serving Chicken (Breast thigh,   1

Or drumstick) (Skin Removed)

Directions

Take all the ingredients except the chicken, and blend them together in a blender. Transfer to a bowl and place it in the refrigerator overnight.

Heat up the grill to approximately 350°F. First dip the chicken pieces into the barbeque sauce and then start grilling. This will take nearly half an hour and you should keep turning the pieces to ensure they are cooked through. Drip the remainder of the barbeque sauce over the pieces as they cook.

Basque Chicken Stew

This ethnic style stew is very tasty and is great for potlucks and gatherings. It can be cooked in large amounts and makes great leftovers. You can easily store it in the refrigerator for nearly three days.

Preparation Time: 15 minutes

Cooking Time: 120 minutes

Serving: 2 ½ cups serving for 4 people

Sodium per Serving: 410 mg

Ingredients

- [ ] Saffron Threads ¼ cup
- [ ] Boiling Water ½ cup
- [ ] Olive Oil 2 tsp
- [ ] Garlic (Sliced) 2 cloves
- [ ] Onion (Sliced into Half Moons)1 large
- [ ] Boneless Skinless Chicken Thighs (Cubed)   1 lb
- [ ] Paprika 2 tsp
- [ ] Salt ½ tsp
- [ ] Fresh Ground Black Pepper (To Taste)
- [ ] No Salt Added Diced Tomatoes1 (15 ounce) can
- [ ] Water 4 cups
- [ ] Lentils 1 cup
- [ ] Green Bell Pepper (Julienned)1 medium

☐ Yellow Bell Pepper (Julienned)1 medium

Directions

Preheat the oven to 325°F and put the saffron threads in a small cup and pour boiling water over them. Set it aside for twenty minutes so that it dissolves and gives off its typical color.

-

Heat the olive oil in a large oven-proof pot, over moderate flame. Fry the garlic for around two minutes. Stir to prevent the garlic from sticking to the bottom of the pot. Next add the onions to the pot and stir fry them for five minutes. Then toss in the chicken and stir fry it for three minutes. It must be light brown when done. One by one add the tomatoes, lentils, peppers and seasonings. Then add the water and stir it well.

Finally add the water with dissolved saffron threads and stir. Cover the pot and place it in the preheated oven. It is advisable that the pot should be a Dutch oven because the pot has to stay in the oven for ninety minutes to two hours. Stir the contents of the pot after twenty minute intervals. Serve while hot.

Black bean Chili

The crackling taste of chilies with black beans warms up the taste buds. It can be served with a variety of things and leftovers can be stored and re-used in whatever way is desired. This recipe can be doubled and tripled.

Preparation Time: 20minutes

Cooking Time: 40 minutes

Serving: 1 ½ cup serving for 6 people

Sodium per Serving: 451 mg

Ingredients

- ☐ Olive Oil 1 tsp
- ☐ Garlic (Sliced) 2 cloves
- ☐ Onion (Diced) 1 large
- ☐ Ground Turkey (Breast in better) 1 ½ lbs
- ☐ Water 6 cups
- ☐ Chili Powder 2 tsp
- ☐ Ground Cumin 1 tsp
- ☐ Salt ¾ tsp
- ☐ Ground Cinnamon   1/8 tsp
- ☐ No Salt Added Black Beans2 (15 ounce) cans
- ☐ Reduced-Fat Cheddar Cheese (Shredded)   3 ounces
- ☐ Cilantro Leaves ½ cup

☐ Reduced Fat Sour Cream6 Tbsp

Heat up the olive oil in a large pan over medium heat and stir fry the garlic in it for around two minutes. Then cook the diced onions for around three to five minutes till they have softened. Then place the ground turkey in the pan and cook it till it has changed color to a light brown.

Sprinkle the salt, pepper, cinnamon, cumin and chili powder over the ground turkey and give it a good stir. Then pop in the black beans and finally add the water bit by bit into the ground turkey and beans. Stir it up and as the chili begins to boil, reduce the heat to low and allow it to simmer. Let it cook for around forty minutes and stir occasionally to make sure the heat is evenly distributed.

When it is time to serve, sprinkle ½ ounce of the cheese, around 1 ½ tablespoon of cilantro leaves and drop a dollop of sour cream on each serving. You can add a cornbread muffin to each serving if you like.

Cashew Chicken

Cashew nuts are sweet and they are quite tasty when combined with chicken. The saucy chicken works well with chicken. This recipe can be doubled, tripled or multiplied by four as per requirements. The leftovers can be kept in the refrigerator for around two days but need to be reheated gently.

Preparation Time: 20minutes

Cooking Time: 40 minutes

Serving: 1 ½ cup s over rice serving for 4 people

Sodium per Serving: 391 mg

Ingredients

☐ Frozen Shelled Edamame (Soy beans)1 cup

☐ Water   2 cups

☐ Brown Rice (Uncooked) 1 cup

☐ Dark Sesame Oil 2 tsp

☐ White Onion (Diced) 1 medium

☐ Garlic (Minced) 1 clove

☐ Boneless Skinless Chicken Breast (Cut into Strips) 1 lb

☐ Raw Cashews ½ cup

☐ Fresh Ginger (Peeled and Minced)1 Tbsp

☐ Low Sodium Chicken or Vegetable Broth½ cup

- [ ] Low-Sodium Soy Sauce 2 Tbsp
- [ ] Maple Syrup 1 Tbsp

Directions

Take the frozen edamame and rinse with cool water and leave in a colander for draining.

You have to boil the water in a medium sized sauce pan and when it reaches boiling point then add the brown rice to it. Once the rice is boiling in it, lower the heat and let it simmer for nearly half an hour. Keep the pan partially covered.

Try not to let all the liquid in the rice dry up and do not stir it while it cooks. During this process, heat up one teaspoon of the sesame oil in a large non stick pan. Cook the diced onions in and keep stirring them till they are soft but not brown. Remove the onions and set them aside.

Add a teaspoon of sesame oil to the pan again and now cook the minced garlic in it. Keep the heat gentle so that the garlic does not burn but stays soft and gives off a lovely aroma. Now add the chicken, nuts and ginger to it. Stir fry the chicken till it change to a white color. This is a signal that you can add the broth, maple syrup and soy sauce to it. Stir it around and then drop the onions back into the pan. Let this cook for around five minutes and stir it occasionally.

The edamame should be thawed by now and can be added to the pan. Cook the mixture for around five to eight minutes. Make sure the chicken gets cooked through. Serve it as a topping over brown rice.

Chicken and Smoked Gouda Pizza

Gouda is a very smooth textured cheese that has a distinct and delightful taste. Using it to top pizza is like adding a luxury to the base. This recipe needs preparation of separate whole wheat pizza dough or you can buy a gluten-free ready to cook crust from the market. It will best to consume the pizza right away because it does not store well. You can multiply it as many times as you want to.

Preparation Time: 40minutes

Cooking Time: 10 minutes

Serving: 1 individual pizza serving for 2 people

Sodium per Serving: 348 mg

Ingredients

☐ Olive Oil 1 tsp

☐ Onion (Sliced) 1 medium

☐ Boneless Skinless Chicken Thighs (Cut into Strips) 6 ounces

☐ Dried Sage 1 tsp

☐ Salt   1/8 tsp

☐ Fresh Ground Black Pepper (To Taste)

☐ Grape Tomatoes (Halved)   2 ounces

☐ Smoked Gouda Cheese (Grated)   1 ½ ounces

☐ Whole Wheat Pizza Dough Recipe (or choose a ½

Gluten-free Pizza Crust)

Preheat the oven to 500°F and place a large baking sheet or pizza stone in it.

Fry the onions for around ten minutes in the olive oil, over moderate heat. The onions should not be over browned in the process and keep stirring. Transfer the onions to a bowl and now coo the chicken thighs in the oil. Increase the heat and sprinkle salt, pepper and sage over the chicken. Cook for seven to ten minutes and add to the bowl with the onions. Combine it with the tomatoes and give it a good tossing.

When the oven is ready, roll out the dough into two individual pizzas. You can freeze any leftover dough by wrapping tightly in plastic wrap. Cover the pizza base with the chicken mixture and sprinkle the smoked Gouda over it.

Pop the pizzas in the oven and bake for around ten minutes. Rotate the pizzas during the baking to cook evenly. The crust should be light brown and crispy when done.

Blackened Redfish | Low Sodium Version

Redfish is a fresh water fish and cooking it right will yield a delicious meal that can be used for entertaining guests or for family. This dish can serve as a good leftover for later use. You can double or triple it easily but you will need a larger cooking utensil for it then.

Preparation Time: 20minutes

Cooking Time: 10 minutes

Serving: 4 ounces of fish serving for 4 people

Sodium per Serving: 346 mg

Ingredients

- ☐ Paprika 2 tsp
- ☐ Salt ½ tsp
- ☐ Onion Powder   ¼ tsp
- ☐ Garlic Powder   ¼ tsp
- ☐ Cayenne Pepper¼ tsp
- ☐ Fresh Ground Black Pepper ¼ tsp
- ☐ Dried Thyme Leaves¼ tsp
- ☐ Dried Oregano Leaves¼ tsp
- ☐ Filets of Red Snapper (4 ounces) 4
- ☐ Spray Olive or grape-seed oil

Directions

First you have to preheat the oven to a very high temperature of 500°F. Then take a heavy cast iron skillet and put it in the oven.

Mix up the seasonings in a small bowl. Place the fish fillet skin side down on a flat surface and first spray it with oil and then coat it with the spice mixture.

Spray some oil on the hot skillet and gently place the fish in it with the skin side facing up. Now put the skillet back in the oven and bake for eight to ten minutes. The fish will have a crisp top and lovely finish.

Baked Cumin Trout with Squash and Pumpkin Seeds | Low Sodium Version

Trout has always been one of the most favored fish when it comes to catching and cooking. It can be coupled with just about anything for an end result that is appealing to the taste buds and to the eyes.

This recipe needs Wild rice for the final serving, so you have to prepare it beforehand or during the cooking of the trout. The recipe can be multiplied up to five times and makes good leftovers that can be used in sandwiches.

Preparation Time: 15minutes

Cooking Time: 150 minutes

Serving: 1 ½ cup of rice and 4 ounces of fish serving for 2 people

Sodium per Serving: 499 mg

Ingredients

☐ Grape-seed Oil 3 tsp

☐ Salt 1/8 tsp

☐ Fresh Ground Black Pepper1/8 tsp

☐ Maple Syrup 2 tsp

☐ Apple Cider Vinegar (Heinz is gluten-free) 1 tsp

☐ Ground Cumin ¾ tsp

☐ Grape-seed Oil 1 tsp

- [ ] Raw Pumpkin Seeds   1 ounce
- [ ] Yellow Squash 8 ounces
- [ ] Filets Fresh Trout (4 ounces)2

Directions

Preheat the oven to 400°F. Then the first three teaspoons of the grape seed oil need to be combined with the salt, black pepper, cumin powder, maple syrup and vinegar. Mix them up in a bowl.

Heat up the remaining grape seed oil in a pan over moderate heat and cook the pumpkin seeds for around five minutes in it. Once the seeds start turning brown, drop the diced squash into the pan.

Cook the squash over moderate heat and keep on stirring until it softens up a bit. Remove it from heat.

Arrange the cooked wild rice in two ovenproof dishes and drip a quarter of the oil and cumin mixture over the trout. Place the dishes in the preheated oven and let the trout cook for around five minutes.

Take the dishes out and drip the remaining oil and cumin mixture over the trout and top off with equal portions of the cooked pumpkin and squash mixture. Return the dishes to the oven and bake for five to seven more minutes. Serve as soon as it is cooked.

Fillet of Grouper with Four Onion Marmalade

<u>The four onion marmalade adds a zingy taste to this fillet but it contains green onions, which can cause problems for people using Coumadin®. So the green onions can be replaced with an extra onion.</u>

Preparation Time: 45minutes

Cooking Time: 15 minutes

Serving: 4 ounces of fish serving for 4 people

Sodium per Serving: 359 mg

Ingredients

- ☐ Bunch Green Onions1
- ☐ Spray Olive Oil
- ☐ Unsalted Butter   1 tsp
- ☐ White Onion (Sliced Thin) 1 medium
- ☐ Red Onion (Sliced Thin)1 medium
- ☐ Shallots (Sliced Thin)2 large
- ☐ Salt ¼ tsp
- ☐ Ground Black Pepper1/8 tsp
- ☐ Maple Syrup   1 tsp
- ☐ Balsamic Vinegar1 Tbsp
- ☐ White Wine   ½ cup
- ☐ Water 1 cup
- ☐ Grouper Filets (4 Ounces) 4

☐ Spray Olive Oil

Preheat oven to a temperature of 325°F. Take a medium sized ovenproof skillet and place it in the oven. Firstly, trim the top green part from the green onions and put them in the preheated skillet after spraying some olive oil on it. It will take around ten minutes to cook them completely and you should turn them once to roast properly on both sides. Remove the pan from the oven. Allow them to cool before chopping them into ½ inch pieces. Do not turn off the oven but increase the heat to 400°F.

Melt the butter in a large non-stick over moderate flame. Now stir fry all the types of onions and the remaining white parts of the green onion. Brown the onions but don't overcook them or let them burn. Sprinkle with the salt and pepper and top off with the maple syrup, water, vinegar and white wine. Boil the mixture and then lower the heat to let it simmer for some time. The liquid should reduce to around 3 tablespoons when it is done.

Put a large ovenproof pan in the preheated oven. Now take half of this mixture and add the scallions to it too. Pop them in a food processor and using pulse action, blend it very carefully till it looks like marmalade. Avoid blending it too much or it will take the consistency of a sauce, which is not desirable.

Take the preheated pan from the oven and spray it with olive oil. Sprinkle the fish with seasonings and place it skin side up on the pan. Pop it in the oven and cook for nearly three minutes before turning the fish and cooking it for seven to ten minutes more. The cooking time depends on the thickness of the fish. Serve with a helping of the onion marmalade.

Fish cakes

This ready to eat kind of recipe is good for quick and on the go meals. Cooked leftovers can be used after 24 hours. You can multiply it up to five times.
Lightly brown the bread in a toaster. Then cool it and chop it in a blender or chopper to make crumbs. Take the fish and roughly chop into smaller bits with the help of a knife. If you wish to use a food processor then use pulse action to prevent it from turning into paste.

Preparation Time: 20minutes

Cooking Time: 15 minutes

Serving: 2 fish cakes serving for 4 people

Sodium per Serving: 342 mg

Ingredients

- ☐ Whole Wheat or gluten-free Bread 2 slices
- ☐ White Fish (like Cod, Tilapia or Halibut) 1 lb
- ☐ Worcestershire Sauce   2 tsp
- ☐ Dijon Mustard 2 tsp
- ☐ Egg 1 large
- ☐ Rib Celery (Diced)   1
- ☐ Grated Lemon Peel   ½ tsp
- ☐ Reduced-Fat Mayonnaise2 Tbsp
- ☐ Dried Thyme ½ tsp
- ☐ Salt 1/8 tsp

☐ Fresh Ground Black pepper (To Taste)

☐ Extra Virgin Olive Oil   2 Tbsp

Directions

Preheat the oven to 325° F. Then in a bowl mix the fold the fish in the breadcrumbs. Top it off with Worcestershire sauce, celery, lemon peel, mayonnaise, egg, mustard, thyme, salt and pepper. Gently fold the fish with the seasoning and sauces, until it is completely blended. Pat the mixture into eight cakes and put them in the refrigerator for chilling.

First you have to fry the cakes in oil. So heat up the oil in a large non-stick pan and keep the heat high. Place the cakes in smoking hot oil but reduce the heat to moderate. Then fry them for three minutes on one and then turn to fry around two minutes on the other side. This will give them a brown finish.

Place the pan in the preheated oven and cook for nearly ten minutes.

-

Garam Masala Scented Risotto with Seared Salmon | Low Sodium Version

This aromatic dish has the Indian touch to it but is very healthy and tasty. Diet conscious people can make it a regular on their menu. This recipe can be multiplied up to five times. You can store leftovers in the refrigerator but reheat them gently.

Preparation Time: 15 minutes

Cooking Time: 15 minutes

Serving: 2 cups risotto with 4 ounces of fish serving for 2 people

Sodium per Serving: 437 mg

Ingredients

- ☐ Olive Oil 1 tsp
- ☐ Garam Masala 1 tsp
- ☐ Onion (Diced) 1 medium
- ☐ Garlic (Minced) 2 cloves
- ☐ Arborio Rice ½ cup
- ☐ Light Coconut Milk ¼ cup
- ☐ Water 2 cups
- ☐ Salt 1/8 tsp
- ☐ Fresh Ground Black Pepper (To Taste)
- ☐ Pepper Jelly 2 Tbsp

- ☐ Low Sodium Chicken or Vegetable Broth 2 Tbsp
- ☐ Spray Olive Oil
- ☐ Salmon Filets (4 ounces)2
- ☐ Parmigiano-Reggiano   1 ounce

Directions

Heat up the olive oil in a non stick pan of medium size. Add garam masala to the pan and stir fry it for nearly two minutes. Then drop in the onions and garlic. Cook the onions till they get lightly limp. Now add the Arborio rice and cook it for around two minutes. Now pour the coconut milk and water into it and sprinkle the seasoning. Stir it and reduce the heat to let the rice simmer. Let it cook for twelve to fifteen minutes. This will soften up the rice.

Preheat the oven to 375°F and place an ovenproof pan in it.

Take the pepper jelly and mix it with the chicken stock. Then when the risotto is nearly ready, then lightly spray the preheated pan with olive oil. Place the fillets skin side down into the pan and pop it back into the oven. Let the fillets cook on one side for five minutes before turning them and adding the pepper jelly sauce to the pan. Cook on this side for three to four minutes. In the meanwhile, drop the cheese into the risotto and stir well.

When serving, place risotto in a bowl and then put the cooked salmon fillet on top. Drip the pepper jelly sauce from the pan over the bowl.

Ginger Papaya White Fish

White fish can be served with a variety of colorful accompaniments to make a nutritious and appealing dish. This recipe can be multiplied as many times as desired but try to consume on the same day as storage is not possible.

Preparation Time: 10minutes

Cooking Time: 15 minutes

Serving: 6 ounces fish serving for 2 people

Sodium per Serving: 384 mg

Ingredients

☐ Sesame Oil 1 tsp

☐ Ground Ginger ½ tsp

☐ Papaya Juice ¼ cup

☐ Salt ¼ tsp

☐ Fresh Ground Black Pepper (To Taste)

☐ Spray Olive Oil

☐ 6 ounce Whitefish Filets (Cod, Orange roughly   2 or Tilapia)

☐ Corn Starch 1 tsp

☐ Water 4 Tbsp

☐ Fresh Cilantro Leaves   2 Tbsp

Directions

Whisk together the sesame oil, ground ginger, salt, pepper and papaya juice. Heat up a non-stick skillet on medium heat and spray it lightly with olive oil. Cook the fish fillets in it for four minutes on each side.

While the fish is cooking, prepare a cornstarch mixture by adding four tablespoons of water to the cornstarch. Blend it properly and then add it slowly to the papaya sauce until it is well blended.

Now pour the papaya sauce over the fish in the pan. Turn the fish one and transfer it to the serving plates. Let the papaya sauce mix up with the liquids from the fish and then pour that over the fillets and sprinkle with cilantro.

Ginger Peanut White Fish

This version of the white fish is also versatile and can be paired with a lot of things to get good results. It can be cooked in larger amounts because leftovers can be used in sandwiches the next day.

Preparation Time: 20minutes

Cooking Time: 10 minutes

Serving: 4 ounces fish serving for 4 people

Sodium per Serving: 217 mg

Ingredients

- ☐ Sesame Oil 4 tsp
- ☐ Garlic (Minced) 1 clove
- ☐ Shallot (Minced) 1 large
- ☐ Raw Unsalted Peanuts (Shelled) ¼ cup
- ☐ Fresh Ginger (Minced) 3 Tbsp
- ☐ Lime (Juiced) ½
- ☐ Sugar ½ tsp
- ☐ Low Sodium Soy or Gluten-free Tamari Sauce 1 Tbsp
- ☐ Fresh Ground Black pepper (To Taste)
- ☐ Low Sodium Chicken Broth 1 cup
- ☐ 4 ounce Whitefish Filets (Halibut, Grouper, Cod) 4

Directions

Heat three teaspoons of the sesame oil over medium heat. Fry the garlic in it for around three minutes and make sure you do not let it burn. Lower the heat if needed. Pop the peanuts and shallots into the pan and cook for three more minutes. Now add the ginger and cook for around five minutes more. Stir in the lime juice, stock and soy sauce and sprinkle pepper over it too.

Cook the sauce for ten minutes and reduce the heat to let it simmer. The sauce should be reduced by half when done. Do not remove from stove but keep the heat at lowest.

In another skillet, fry the fish in the remaining sesame oil. Make sure to add the fish only when the oil has heated up. Fry the fish for around five minutes on each side. Top the fish with the sauce when serving.

-

Grilled Halibut with Tangerines and Capers

<u>This recipe can be multiplied as many times as you want and you can use the leftover in sandwiches later on.</u>

Preparation Time: 10 minutes

Cooking Time: 20 minutes

Serving: 4 ounces fish serving for 2 people

Sodium per Serving: 439 mg

Ingredients

☐ Shallot (Minced)   1 small

☐ Garlic (Minced) 1 clove

☐ Tangerine (Peeled, Seeded and separated 1

☐ into sections)

☐ Olive Oil 2 Tbsp

☐ Caper Juice 2 tsp

☐ Capers 2 tsp

☐ Salt ¼ tsp

☐ Fresh Ground Black Pepper (To Taste)

☐ Cilantro Leaves 1 Tbsp

☐ Halibut Filets (4 ounce)   2

☐ Spray Olive Oil

Directions

Take a small bowl and toss together the garlic, tangerine, shallot, caper liquid, capers, salt, pepper, olive oil and cilantro. Refrigerate them to chill.

Next take a large non-stick frying pan and put over high heat. Once it has heated up, spray with the oil and lay out the halibut fillets on it. Cook for six to eight minutes on each side and the halibut should be done in roughly fifteen minutes.

Serve it with the chilled tangerine mixture.

-

Grilled Red Snapper with Garlic Tartar Sauce

The Red Snapper family of fish has a flesh that can be complimented with the flavors of garlic and tartar. This recipe needs the preparation of Garlic Tartar Sauce separately. It can be multiplied up to five times and the leftovers can be used later on in sandwiches.

Preparation Time: 10 minutes

Cooking Time: 10 minutes

Serving: 4 ounces fish serving for 2 people

Sodium per Serving: 423 mg

Ingredients

- ☐ Filets of Red Snapper (4 ounce)2
- ☐ Salt 1/8 tsp
- ☐ Fresh Ground Black Pepper
- ☐ Spray Grape-seed or Olive Oil
- ☐ Garlic Tartar Sauce   2 Tbsp

Directions

You can use either the grill or a grill pan so heat up the grill or place a large grill pan in the oven at 375°F.
Rinse the fish fillet with water and then pat them dry. Lay out flat on a cutting board and poke the skin with a knife after half inch. Do no cut deeper than the skin and season with the salt and pepper.
When the grill or oven has heated up to the right temperature, spray lightly with oil and put the fish skin

side down on the grill. Let it cook for five minutes before turning it and cooking the other side for around three minutes.
Serve with the prepared Garlic and Tartar Sauce.

Grouper with Caramelized Shallot Horseradish Sauce

This recipe can be multiplied up to four times and makes good leftovers that can be utilized in sandwiches.

Preparation Time: 45 minutes

Cooking Time: 15 minutes

Serving: 4 ounces fish serving for 4 people

Sodium per Serving: 439 mg

Ingredients

- ☐ Shallots 8 ounces
- ☐ Spray Grape-seed or Olive Oil
- ☐ White Wine   ¼ cup
- ☐ Salt ¼ tsp
- ☐ Fresh Ground Black Pepper
- ☐ Prepared Horseradish2 tsp
- ☐ Honey 1 tsp
- ☐ Grouper Filets (4 ounce) 4

Directions

For this recipe you will need a non-reactive utensil for the cooking, like a stainless steel pan. Preheat the oven to 375°F and place the shallots in the pan. Spray lightly with oil and cover it. Then pop the pan in the preheated oven and allow the shallots to roast for half an hour. At half time take the pan out and give the shallots a good tossing.

After the half hour is up, pour white wine over the shallots and season with salt and pepper. Cook for fifteen more minutes in the oven. Finally take out the pan and let it cool for five minutes.

Blend the shallots with the horseradish and honey in a blender or chopper. You should get a smooth puree.

Place an oven proof skillet in the oven and raise the temperature to 426°F. Once the pan is hot enough, spray the pan with grape seed oil and lay out the grouper fillets in it. Pop it back into the oven and let it cook for five to six minutes. Then turn the fish and drip around 3 tablespoons of sauce over each fillet. Cook this side for around five to seven minutes more. Serve straight from the oven.

Grouper with Horseradish Glaze

Preparation Time: 10 minutes

Cooking Time: 15 minutes

Serving: 4 ounces fish serving for 2 people

Sodium per Serving: 466 mg

Ingredients

- ☐ Olive Oil   1 tsp
- ☐ Garlic (Sliced Thin)2 clove
- ☐ Prepared Horseradish3 tsp
- ☐ Fresh Thyme Leaves2 tsp
- ☐ Lemon (Juiced)   1
- ☐ Maple Syrup   2 tsp
- ☐ Salt ¼ tsp
- ☐ Unsalted Butter   2 Tbsp
- ☐ Fresh Ground Black Pepper (To Taste)
- ☐ Spray Olive Oil or Grape-seed Oil
- ☐ Grouper Filets (4 ounce) 2

Directions

Place an oven proof skillet in the oven and preheat it to the temperature of 400°F. Pour olive oil into a small pan and place it on moderate heat. Fry the garlic in it for around three to five minutes. Keep stirring and do not let the garlic burn. Now pour lemon juice and maple syrup over it. Season with salt and thyme and add the horseradish. Lower the heat slightly and cook for around five more minutes. Now drop the spread into the pan and sprinkle the black pepper too. Stir it until the spread melts and then remove from heat. Take the preheated pan and spray lightly with oil. Now lay out the grouper skin side up. Pop it back into the oven and bake for six minutes before turning it and adding the sauce to the pan. Cook for five more minutes on this side and then remove from the oven. When serving the fish, drip the sauce from the pan over it.

Healthy Asian Beef with Broccoli

Beef is not just a good source of protein but also a very flavorsome kind of meat. Health conscious people argue that it is not good for health but in small amounts and with the right accompaniments, it can be served as a wonderful part of any meal.

This recipe can be multiplied as many times as you want and you can keep the leftovers in the refrigerator. It also works well with brown rice.

Preparation Time: 10 minutes

Cooking Time: 20 minutes

Serving: 2 cups serving for 2 people

Sodium per Serving: 415 mg

Ingredients

☐ Dark Sesame Oil or Canola Oil2 tsp

☐ Fresh Ginger (Peeled and Minced) 1 Tbsp

☐ Onion (Sliced) 1 large

☐ Top Round or Other Stew Meat (thinly Sliced) 8 ounces

☐ Broccoli Flowerets   8 ounces

☐ Hoisin Sauce 2 Tbsp

☐ Chinese or Dijon Mustard1 tsp

☐ Fresh Ground Black Pepper (To Taste)

☐ Low Sodium Chicken or Vegetable Broth ½ cup

□ Cornstarch 1 ½ tsp

□ Cold Water 2 Tbsp

Directions

Heat up the sesame oil in a deep pan or wok and cook the ginger and onion in it. Stir frequently to prevent burning and even cooking. The onions should get soft. Now pop in the beef and stir fry for about three minutes. The beef should turn light brown. Reduce heat and toss together with the broccoli. Cover the pan and let it cook for five minutes. Stir every now and then.

Pour the hoisin sauce into the pan and add the pepper and mustard as well. Mix well and let it cook for five minutes more. Then stir in the stock.

Prepare the cornstarch mixture by adding the cornstarch to the cold water and stirring till dissolved. Slowly add the cornstarch mixture to the pan and stir. Remove from heat and stir for a while. Serve with brown rice preferably.

Asparagus Linguine

This recipe can be multiplied up to five times but try to consume it within one day, because it does not make good leftovers.

Preparation Time: 15 minutes

Cooking Time: 25 minutes

Serving: 2ounces pasta serving for 2 people

Sodium per Serving: 561 mg

Ingredients

☐ Spears Asparagus (Steamed until al dente) 6 ounces

☐ Water 1 quart

☐ 2% Milk ½ cup

☐ Flour 1 Tbsp

☐ Extra Virgin Olive Oil 1 tsp

☐ Garlic (Minced) 2 cloves

☐ Fresh Lemon Juice 2 Tbsp

☐ Onion (Minced) 1 small

☐ Semi Soft Goat Cheese 2 ounces

☐ Salt 1/8 tsp

☐ Tomato (Peeled, Seeded and Chopped) 1 small

☐ Fresh Basil 1 Tbsp

☐ Parmigiano-Reggiano (Grated)1 ounce

☐ Linguine 4 ounces

☐ Water 4 quarts

Directions

Take a quart of water in a shallow saucepan and heat it over medium to high heat. Take it to poaching stage which is just before boiling. Then blanch the asparagus spears in it for six to eight minutes. The spears will soften and turn bright green, once they are done. Remove from pan and arrange four spears in both the bowls.

Take a mixing cup and mix together the milk and flour until it becomes a smooth mixture without clumps.

Now heat up the olive oil in a sauté pan, over a moderate flame and cook the minced garlic. Do not let it change color and only soften it, then pour the lemon juice over it. Now stir it till the juice is almost gone. Now add the onions to it too. Keep cooking and once the onion is limp and loses its color, reduce the heat. Stir in the milk mixture and whisk it as the sauce thickens. Season with salt and then add the cheese. Lower the heat to minimum and continue whisking till the cheese has melted completely. Now remove from heat.

Preheat the oven to 350°F. Chop up the fresh basil and mix it up with the tomatoes. Boil four quarts of water in a stock pot and then add the linguine. Cook it for around fifteen minutes till it is firm but chewable. Drain

<u>from the pot and add to the sauté pan into the sauce.
Toss the pasta in it to coat with the sauce.</u>

Switch the oven to broil and now place the coated pasta on top of the asparagus spears in the serving bowls. Sprinkle the tomato basil mixture and shredded cheese over the bowls. Place under the broiler and bake till the cheese has melted. Then the asparagus linguine is ready to be served.

Baked Penne

Penne pasta has the ability to retain any sauce or salad that it is served with, so it can be fun to change the condiments with it. This recipe can be doubled or tripled and leftovers can be stored in the refrigerator or frozen in tightly sealed plastic bags.

Preparation Time: 20 minutes

Cooking Time: 30 minutes

Serving: 2.67 ounces pasta serving for 6 people

Sodium per Serving: 300 mg

Ingredients

- [ ] Yellow Bell Pepper1 large
- [ ] Red Bell Peppers2 large
- [ ] Eggplant (Cut into 1 inch Cubes) 1 lb
- [ ] Flat Leaf Parsley (Coarsely chopped) ¼ cup
- [ ] Fresh Oregano (Coarsely chopped) 2 Tbsp
- [ ] Pecorino-Romano (Grated) 1 ounce
- [ ] Salt ¼ tsp
- [ ] Pepper to Taste
- [ ] Unsalted Butter 2 tsp
- [ ] Fontina Cheese (Shredded) 3 ounces

Directions

Preheat the oven to 375°F. Deseed the peppers and dice them into small squares. Spray an ovenproof pan with olive oil and add the eggplant, peppers and shallots to it. Now pop the pan into the preheated oven and let the vegetables roast for around fifteen to twenty minutes.

During the roasting, boil five quarts of water in a deep stock pot and cook the penne pasta for around 15 minutes in it. Drain the pasta when it is still firm and seems slightly underdone.

In a large glass bowl or stainless steel bowl, mix together the Romano cheese, egg substitute, parsley, salt, oregano and pepper. Toss in the penne pasta and the butter. Keep on tossing till the pasta has gotten completely coated with the ingredients. Now add the roasted vegetables to the penne and fold them in.

Spray a twelve inches oblong baking dish with olive oil and arrange the penne mixture into it. Sprinkle the grated fontina over the dish and pop it in the preheated oven for fifteen to twenty minutes. The top should be slightly brown when the penne is baked.

Butternut Squash Risotto

Preparation Time: 20 minutes

Cooking Time: 30 minutes

Serving: 2 cups serving for 4 people

Sodium per Serving: 460 mg

Ingredients

- [ ] Butternut Squash   2 lbs
- [ ] Spray Olive Oil
- [ ] Extra Virgin Olive Oil   2 tsp
- [ ] Leek 1 large
- [ ] Red Onion (Diced)   ½ medium
- [ ] Arborio Rice 1 cup
- [ ] Water 3 cup
- [ ] Low Sodium Chicken or Vegetable Broth 1 cup
- [ ] Dry Sherry ¼ cup
- [ ] Salt ¼ tsp
- [ ] Fresh Ground Black Pepper
- [ ] Ground Paprika ¼ tsp
- [ ] Parmigiano-Reggiano (Grated)1 ½ ounces
- [ ] Italian Parsley Leaves   ½ cup

Directions

Preheat the oven to 325°F. Place the squash on a cutting board and cut it lengthwise. Deseed the

123

squash. Now take a baking sheet and place the squash cut side up on it. Spray it with olive oil and place it in the preheated oven. Let the squash roast for almost an hour. It will be slightly soft. Take it out of the oven and allow it to cool. There will be the squash juices in the cavity part. Once it has cooled, drain away the liquid and once again put the squash on the board. Carefully peel off the skin and cut into three long slices. Keep the slices in place like the shape of the squash and now slice them into thinner sections by cutting lengthwise after ¼ inch and then cut the slices horizontally after ¼ inch. This will yield ½ cubes. Set these cubes aside.

Now it is the leek's turn. Chop of its root and first of all slice it in half to get a green top and white bottom. Rinse the green part with water and chop it very finely. Next take the white part and cut very thin long slices. Clean them too.

Quickly heat up the olive oil in a large saucepan and drop in the green half of the leek into it. Lower the heat to moderate and stir fry slowly. When the green appears to be wilted, add the white part and diced onion. Lower the heat even more and cook for around five minutes. Add the rice and stir the mixture for three more minutes before adding stock, sherry, two cups of water and season with salt and pepper. Cook the rice on moderately high heat and stir regularly. Then slowly add the rest of the water to the pan.

Sprinkle paprika over the rice and keep on cooking. The total time taken will be around twenty to twenty-five minutes and you might have to add some more water. Do not let the rice get mushy and leave some of the saucy liquid in it. Stir in the cheese and let it melt before folding in the squash and topping off with parsley.

Serve hot.

Chalupas | Low Sodium Version

This on the go kind of meal is very appetizing and easy to make. You do need Refried Black Beans and Guacamole, which can be prepared beforehand. Do not try to store the assembled chalupas because they tend to become crumbly and fall apart easily. You can multiply the recipe as many times as you want to.

Preparation Time: 10 minutes

Cooking Time: 10 minutes

Serving: 3 chalupas serving for 2 people

Sodium per Serving: 405 mg

Ingredients

☐ Soft Corn Tortillas   6

☐ Refried Black Beans (Dr. Gourmet Recipe) ½ cup

☐ Reduced Fat Monterey Jack Cheese (Shredded)   2 ounces

☐ Leaves Romaine Lettuce (Shredded fine) 6

☐ Tomato (Coarsely chopped)1 large

☐ Cilantro Leaves (Chopped)½ cup

☐ Guacamole (Dr. Gourmet Recipe) 6 Tbsp

☐ Fresh Ground Black Pepper (to taste)

Directions

Preheat the oven to 375°F and then lay out the six tortillas on a baking sheet. Equally divide the refried beans between all the tortillas and sprinkle some cheese over each. Place the tray in the preheated oven and bake long enough to melt the cheese.

Remove the tray from the oven and serve the tortillas with tomato, lettuce, pepper, guacamole, cilantro and salsa.

Vegetarian Corn and Black Bean Taco Salad

Cooking purely vegetarian meals can be challenging since they require imagination and appealing flavors. This recipe is good for all kinds of eating styles and the corn and black bean mixture can be stored for around two days.

Preparation Time: 10 minutes

Cooking Time: 20 minutes

Serving: 1 large salad serving for 2 people

Sodium per Serving: 521 mg

Ingredients

- ☐ Olive Oil 1 tsp
- ☐ Onion (Diced) 1 medium
- ☐ Green Bell Pepper (Diced)   1 medium
- ☐ Chili Powder ½ tsp
- ☐ Cumin   ½ tsp
- ☐ Salt   ¼ tsp
- ☐ Ear Corn (Kernels cut from Cob)   1
- ☐ No Salt added Black Beans (Drained and Rinsed) 1 (15 ounces) can
- ☐ Water   ¼ cup
- ☐ Unsalted Corn Tortilla Chips   2 ounces
- ☐ Iceberg Lettuce (Sliced thin)   3 cups

- [ ] Tomato (Sliced into small Wedges)1 large
- [ ] Reduced Fat Monterey Jack Cheese (Shredded) 2 ounces
- [ ] Reduced Fat Sour Cream   2 Tbsp

Directions

Heat oil over moderate heat and cook the diced onions in it. Keep stirring till the onions turn soft and then pop in the green bell peppers, cumin, chili powder and salt. Cook till the peppers soften.

The next ingredient to go into the skillet is the corn and you have to cook that for around three minutes too. Now pour the water into it and put the beans in. Cook for around ten minutes and remove from heat when the water has almost disappeared. Now let it cool and refrigerate.

When the bean mixture has chilled, take it out of the refrigerator and start making the salad. In a large bowl sprinkle the taco chips to cover the bottom of the bowl. Then spread the shredded lettuce over it and then the bean mixture. Ring the tomato wedges around the edge of the bowl and top off with the shredded cheese. Finally drop the sour cream over the whole salad and serve.

Corn Quesadilla

This recipe can be multiplied up to five times.

Preparation Time: 20 minutes

Cooking Time: 20 minutes

Serving: 1 quesadilla serving for 2 people

Sodium per Serving: 350 mg

Ingredients

- ☐ Olive Oil 1 tsp
- ☐ Pablano Chili (Seeded and Diced)¼
- ☐ Ear Corn (Shave Kernels from the Cob)1
- ☐ Green Onions (Sliced Crosswise) 2
- ☐ Red Bell Pepper (Seeded and Julienned)½ medium
- ☐ Ground Cumin ¼ tsp
- ☐ Chili Powder 1 tsp
- ☐ Salt 1/8 tsp
- ☐ Fresh Ground Black Pepper (to taste)
- ☐ Water ½ cup
- ☐ Fresh Cilantro Leaves (Chopped)2 Tbsp
- ☐ Spray Oil
- ☐ Corn Tortillas 4
- ☐ Reduced-Fat Monterey Jack Cheese (Shredded) 2 ounces

Directions

Take a large frying pan and heat up the olive oil in it. Cook the poblano in it for three minutes. Then add the corn and cook while tossing frequently. Increase the heat a bit. The kernels should be brown when you add the green onions and red peppers to the pan. Keep cooking this for three minutes and then season with salt, pepper, cumin and chili powder. Stir and cook for two more minutes, then add water. Cook for around ten minutes or till the water has evaporated. Then turn of the heat and add the cilantro. Mix up the vegetables to evenly distribute the spices.

Heat a non-stick griddle pan over moderately high flame and spray it lightly with oil. And place two tortillas in the pan and start layering them. The first layer is ¼ of the cheese on each tortilla and the next layer is ½ of the corn mixture for each tortilla. The final layer is the remaining cheese and then covers each tortilla with another tortilla. Spray a thin film of oil over the finished quesadilla and cook for five minutes on each side. Make sure to press the quesadilla down to make the layers stick together with the melted cheese.

Cream of Potato Soup with Roasted Garlic |

Low Sodium Version

Soups can be served as entrees or simply served with salads for making a complete light meal. You will have to make roasted garlic separately. This recipe can be multiplied up to six times and can be stored.

Preparation Time: 10 minutes

Cooking Time: 50 minutes

Serving: 2 cups serving for 4 people

Sodium per Serving: 422 mg

Ingredients

☐ Olive Oil (Serve with Cole Slaw or Zucchini Salad 1 tsp

☐ White Onion (Diced) 1 small

☐ Idaho Potato (Peeled and Cubed)12 ounces

☐ Water 4 cups

☐ 2% Milk 1 cup

☐ Bulb Roasted Garlic 1

☐ Salt ¼ tsp

☐ Fresh Ground Black Pepper (to taste)

☐ Yukon Gold Potato (Peeled and Cubed)12 ounces

☐ Smoked Gouda (Shredded) 4 ounces

Directions

Cook the onions in moderately heated olive oil for around four minutes. Do not let the onions turn brown. Add the Idaho potato and water. Lower the heat and let the potatoes simmer for half an hour. This will soften up the potatoes.

Transfer the potatoes to a blender and blend together with the milk, roasted garlic and salt and pepper. Once done, put the puree back into the pot. You could use a hand-held blender and puree the ingredients in the pot.

Next addition into the soup is the Yukon gold potatoes and they have to be cooked for around twenty minutes, in order to soften the potatoes.

Serve the soup while it is still hot and sprinkle an ounce of smoked Gouda over each soup bowl.

Creamy Mac and Cheese

Mac and cheese is a favorite among kids and adults alike. It is easy to make but it contains a lot of calories. This recipe is crafted to keep check on the fat and calories! It can be served with a variety of things to add flavor. This recipe can be multiplied up to four times and can be stored though it tends to get all sludge-like. So dilute it a bit with 2% milk when reheating.

Preparation Time: 10 minutes

Cooking Time: 40 minutes

Serving: 2 ounces pasta serving for 4 people

Sodium per Serving: 344 mg

Ingredients

- ☐ Water 4 quarts
- ☐ Whole Wheat Penne Pasta 8 ounces
- ☐ Eggs 2 large
- ☐ 2% Milk (1% Milk will work) ½ cup
- ☐ Reduced-Fat Cheddar Cheese (Grated)   5 ounces
- ☐ Salt 1/8 tsp
- ☐ Fresh Ground Black Pepper

Directions

Quickly boil the water in a stock pot and cook the pasta till it is firm but still chewy.

During the pasta's boiling, whisk together the eggs and milk and transfer it to a deep saucepan. Season with salt and add the cheese to it.

Drain the pasta when it is done and then toss it into the saucepan with the cheese. Cook it over medium heat and keep stirring till the cheese has melted. This will yield a creamy sauce. Cook only till the sauce is very thick and then remove from heat. Season with black pepper and serve after stirring it.

Curried Cauliflower

This Asian style curried cauliflower has an assortment of ingredients and seasonings that can be served with any kind of rice. This recipe can be doubled and tripled if you want to and you can save the leftovers.

Preparation Time: 5 minutes

Cooking Time: 25 minutes

Serving: 1 cup serving for 3 people

Sodium per Serving: 298 mg

Ingredients

☐ Olive Oil 1 tsp

☐ Curry Powder 1 tsp

☐ Ground Cumin ½ tsp

☐ 10 ounce Package Frozen Cauliflower 1

☐ No Salt Added Diced Tomatoes1 (15 ounce) can

☐ Salt ¼ tsp

☐ Fresh Ground Black Pepper (to taste)

☐ No Salt Added Chick Peas (Garbanzos) 1 (15 ounce) can

☐ 2% Milk ¼ cup

☐ Frozen Peas ½ cup

Directions

Fry the cumin and curry powder in the olive oil over moderate heat. Stir well to prevent burning. Once the pan gets hot, fry the onions and cauliflower in it for around five to seven minutes before you drop in the tomatoes and season with salt and pepper. Stir the vegetables for five more minutes.

Now pour the milk into the pan and add the chick peas. Let this cook for seven minutes approximately. The final ingredients are the peas and cook five more minutes after their addition.

Curried Eggplant

This curry has all the exotic Indian spices and tingles the taste buds with the wonderful taste. You can make a large amount of this curry by multiplying it up to five times. Leftovers can be utilized later on.

Preparation Time: 10 minutes

Cooking Time: 30 minutes

Serving: 6 ounces serving for 3 people

Sodium per Serving: 268 mg

Ingredients

- ☐ Olive Oil 1 tsp
- ☐ Curry Powder 2 tsp
- ☐ Ground Coriander 1 tsp
- ☐ Ground Cumin ½ tsp
- ☐ Red Pepper Flakes (Optional) 1/8 tsp
- ☐ Onion (Diced) 1 small
- ☐ Garlic (Sliced) 1 clove
- ☐ Diced Tomatoes 1 (15 ounce) can
- ☐ Salt ¼ tsp
- ☐ Fresh Ground Black Pepper (to taste)
- ☐ Spray Olive Oil
- ☐ Eggplant (Sliced into rounds about ¼ inch thick) 1 ½ lb

☐ Dried Pumpkin Seeds ¼ cup

☐ Paneer Cheese (Cut into small cubes)4 ounces

Directions

Fry the cumin, coriander, cayenne and curry powder in the olive oil over moderate heat. Stir well and do not let the oil get smoking hot. Cook for nearly three minutes. Once the pan gets hot, fry the onions and garlic in it for around five minutes before you drop in the tomatoes and season with salt and pepper. Stir the mixture for ten more minutes and then remove from the pan and puree it with the help of a blender. Set it aside once it is smooth.

Wipe the pan clean and once again heat it up over moderately high heat. Spray the pan with olive oil and cook the eggplant slice in it. Turn the sides until slightly brown on both sides. Keep the pan oiled to prevent the slices from sticking to the pan. Remove from the pan and pat them dry on paper towels.

Preheat the oven to 325°F and prepare a medium sized baking dish (preferably Pyrex) by lining it with aluminum foil. Lay down a layer of the cooked eggplant in the bottom of the dish and pour ½ of the curry paste over it. Then sprinkle half of the pumpkin seeds over it. Proceed with the second layer in the same manner. Then pop the dish in the preheated oven and bake without any cover for ten minutes.

Now take out the dish and sprinkle cheese on top as a final layer and return to the oven. Let it bake till the cheese has melted, which will take only five minutes.

Curried Lentils | Low Sodium Version

Lentils are a good source of protein and do not come with the disadvantages of meat, which is the chief source of protein. Curried lentils are more inclined towards the Indian Thali style and can be served with Indian chapattis or rice. This recipe can be multiplied up to four times and leftovers can be stored.

Preparation Time: 5 minutes

Cooking Time: 30 minutes

Serving: 2 cups serving for 4 people

Sodium per Serving: 420 mg

Ingredients

- ☐ Olive Oil 1 tsp
- ☐ Onion (Diced) 1 medium
- ☐ Carrots (Peeled and Diced)2
- ☐ Ribs Celery (Diced)   2
- ☐ Ground Cumin 1 tsp
- ☐ Curry Powder 1 ½ tsp
- ☐ Low Sodium Chicken or Vegetable Broth 1 cup
- ☐ Water 3 ½ cups
- ☐ Red Lentils 1 cup
- ☐ Raw Pistachios (Shelled)   1/3 cup

- [ ] Raisins 1/3 cup
- [ ] Salt ½ tsp
- [ ] Fresh Ground Black Pepper (to taste)
- [ ] Paneer (Cut into ½ inch cubes)8 ounces
- [ ] Fresh Baby Spinach Leaves8 ounces

Directions

Take a large skillet or pot and heat up the olive oil in it. Cook the onions over moderately high heat for three minutes. Then add the celery and carrots to the onions. Keep stir frying for a further three minutes.

Sprinkle the cumin and curry powder over the pot and cook for one more minute. Finally pour the chicken broth and water into the pot and add the lentils, pistachios, raisins and salt and pepper. Keep cooking the lentils for around ten to fifteen minutes.

A couple of minutes before removing from heat add the paneer to the lentils and let it cook. When serving, arrange spinach leaves in four serving bowls and top with the lentils.

Eggplant Curry with Rice Noodles

Eggplant can be tricky to cook but making a curry from it can preserve its taste and nutritious value. This dish should be consumed within the day since you can't store any leftovers. The recipe can be multiplied up to four times.

Preparation Time: 10 minutes

Cooking Time: 20 minutes

Serving: 1 ½ ounces noodles and veggies serving for 2 people

Sodium per Serving: 479 mg

Ingredients

☐ Olive Oil 1 tsp

☐ Onion (Sliced) 1 small

☐ Crimini Mushrooms (quartered)   4 ounces

☐ Carrot (Peeled and Cubed)   1 large

☐ Eggplant (about ½ pound) (cut into large cubes) 1

☐ Curry Powder 1 tsp

☐ Light Coconut Milk ¼ cup

☐ Salt   1/8 tsp

☐ Sugar   ½ tsp

☐ Water   1 ¾ cup

☐ Fresh Ground Black Pepper (to taste)

- [ ] Raisins   1/3 cup
- [ ] Paneer Cheese (Cubed) 3 ounces
- [ ] Rice Noodles 3 ounces

Directions

In a small bowl, whisk together the coconut milk, salt, pepper, sugar, water and curry powder. Set it aside.

Then heat up the olive oil over moderately high heat. Use a non stick skillet that has a lid or use a pot. Cook the onions in the oil for around two minutes. Then drop in the carrot, mushrooms and eggplant. Give the ingredients a good stir. Cover the pot and lower the heat to medium. Cook the eggplant till it is soft and it will take around six to eight minutes.

Now add the already prepared curry mixture and raisins. Mix it up and then add the rice noodles. Cook it for five more minutes before adding the paneer and covering it up again. Let it cook till the noodles are done that is approximately five minutes.

Eggplant Risotto

Eggplants can give the risotto a very creamy kind of texture. You can multiply this recipe as many times as you want to and you can keep the leftovers for later use.

Preparation Time: 10 minutes

Cooking Time: 20 minutes

Serving: 2 cups serving for 2 people

Sodium per Serving: 482 mg

Ingredients

- ☐ Olive Oil 1 tsp
- ☐ Garlic (Sliced) 1 clove
- ☐ Onion (Sliced) 1 small
- ☐ Eggplant (cut into 1 inch cubes)   1 large
- ☐ Dried Tarragon ¼ tsp
- ☐ Dried Oregano ½ tsp
- ☐ Dried Basil ½ tsp
- ☐ Dried Rosemary ½ tsp
- ☐ Arborio Rice ½ cup
- ☐ Fresh Ground Black Pepper (to taste)
- ☐ Water   3 cups
- ☐ Cherry or Grape Tomatoes   4 ounces
- ☐ Parmigiano-Reggiano (grated)   1 ounce

☐ Fresh Mozzarella (cut into small dice)2 ounces

Directions

Fry the garlic and onion in moderately heated olive oil, for around a minute. While stirring frequently, add the eggplant to the skillet. You can adjust the heat according to cooking speed of the eggplant. Do not burn it but let it turn brown.

Now sprinkle the dried tarragon, oregano, basil and rosemary over the eggplant and add the Arborio rice. Stir it around for a minute and then add the water, pepper and tomatoes. Mix it up well and then let it simmer over reduced heat. Keep up the cooking till the rice is tender and that will take approximately fifteen minutes.

Finally add the parmesan cheese and allow it to blend. When the risotto is ready to be served, top it off with cubed fresh mozzarella.

Fettuccine Alfredo

The creamy Alfredo Sauce is great for all occasions but it is a bit heavy on the digestive system. Those who suffer from digestive disorders like GERD should substitute plain fettuccine with gluten-free or whole wheat pasta.

Preparation Time: 10 minutes

Cooking Time: 20 minutes

Serving: 2 ounces serving for 2 people

Sodium per Serving: 341 mg

Ingredients

- ☐ Extra Virgin Oil1 tsp
- ☐ Garlic (Minced)2 cloves
- ☐ All Purpose White Flour 2 tsp
- ☐ 2% Milk   ¾ cup
- ☐ Semi-soft Goat Cheese 1 ounce
- ☐ Parmigiano-Reggiano (grated)   1 ounce
- ☐ Water   4 quarts
- ☐ Fettuccine4 ounces
- ☐ Flat Leaf Parsley (Minced)   2 Tbsp

Directions

Quickly boil the water in a stock pot and cook the pasta till it is firm but still chewy. This should take around fifteen minutes

During the pasta's boiling, lightly brown the minced garlic in olive oil over moderate heat. Stir it and don't let it get dark brown. Now add the flour into the pan and stir it to blend the oil and flour into a crumbly mixture. Let it cook for a minute then add cold milk bit by bit, whisking hard to prevent clumps from forming. Once the milk is blended in, add the goat cheese to the sauce. Let that melt before adding the Parmigiano-Reggiano cheese to the pan. When the cheese melts, the final result should be a smooth thick paste.

Drain the pasta when it is done and then toss it into the saucepan with the sauce. Then top with a shiver of minced fresh parsley before serving.

Fettuccine with Olive Oil and Garlic

This recipe can be multiplied up to five times but cannot be stored in the refrigerator.

Preparation Time: 10 minutes

Cooking Time: 20 minutes

Serving: 2 ounces serving for 2 people

Sodium per Serving: 465 mg

Ingredients

☐ Water 2 quarts

☐ Whole Wheat or Gluten-free Fettuccine 4 ounces

☐ Extra Virgin Olive Oil   1 Tbsp

☐ Garlic (Minced) 3 cloves

☐ Pitted Black Olives – like Kalamata 6 large

Coarsely Chopped)

☐ White Wine ¼ cup

☐ Salt 1/8 tsp

☐ Fresh Ground Black Pepper (to taste)

☐ Tomatoes (Seeded and cut into strips) 2 medium

☐ Fresh Basil Leaves (chiffonade)8 large

☐ Parmigiano-Reggiano (grated)1 ounce

Directions

Boil water in a large stock pot and put the fettuccine in. Let it cook.

While the pasta cooks, heat up one tablespoon of olive oil in a large skillet over moderate flame. Stir fry the minced garlic and olives in it. Reduce the flame to prevent the garlic from browning too much. When the pasta is done, transfer it to the skillet after draining it. Then increase the heat and pour the white wine in and season with salt and pepper. Toss everything together as the liquid in the pan starts evaporating then toss the tomatoes in and drip the rest of the olive oil over it.

Cook for a few more minutes and mix up the basil into it. When serving the pasta, sprinkle shredded cheese over it.

Fettuccine with Roasted Eggplant and Broccoli

Preparation Time: 20 minutes

Cooking Time: 40 minutes

Serving: 2 ounces serving for 2 people

Sodium per Serving: 388 mg

Ingredients

- ☐ 8 Ounces Eggplants 2
- ☐ Broccoli   8 ounces
- ☐ Water   3 quarts
- ☐ Spray Olive Oil
- ☐ Whole Wheat or Gluten-free Fettuccine4 ounces
- ☐ Olive Oil 1 Tbsp
- ☐ Garlic (Minced) 1 clove
- ☐ Pine-nuts 1 Tbsp
- ☐ Lemon Zest 1 tsp
- ☐ Balsamic Vinegar 2 Tbsp
- ☐ Salt   ¼ tsp
- ☐ Fresh Ground Black Pepper
- ☐ Flat Leaf Parsley 2 Tbsp
- ☐   Aged Gruyere (Asiago or other hard cheese will do) 1 ounce

Directions

Preheat the oven to 325° F and heat up an ovenproof grill pan or sauté pan in it. Break up the broccoli into flowerets having long stems and cut up the eggplant into cubes of one inch each.

You have to steam the eggplant and broccoli. It would be great if you had a steamer but if you do not have one then you can make a steamer yourself! Take a steamer basket and put the vegetables in it. Fit the basket into a deep pan that has the water ready in the bottom. Put the pan over high heat and allow the water to start boiling. Then steam the vegetables for nearly seven minutes.

Remove the vegetables once they are done and let them cool. Take out the preheated pan from the oven and spray it with olive oil. Put the broccoli in it and pop the pan back into the oven for seven to ten minutes. Take it out and remove the broccoli from the pan. Now spray with olive oil again and add the eggplant to it. Now roast it for nearly forty minutes.

When the eggplant has been in the oven for half an hour, boil water in a large stock pot and put the fettuccine in. Let it cook. Then heat up the olive oil over moderate heat and stir fry the garlic, lemon zest and pine nuts. Cook for nearly three minutes.

Once the fettuccine is done, drain it but reserve 1/3 cup of the pasta's liquid. Add the fettuccine to the frying pan and pour vinegar over it. Season with salt and pepper. Add the reserved pasta liquid and add the now roasted broccoli and eggplant. Toss the pasta with the vegetables for two minutes and sprinkle parsley leaves to it.

When serving, grate the aged gruyere over each bowl.

Fettuccine with Roasted Mushrooms and Cipollini Onions

This recipe can be multiplied up to four times but try to consume it within one day because leftovers can't be stored.

Preparation Time: 10 minutes

Cooking Time: 30 minutes

Serving: 2 ounces serving for 3 people

Sodium per Serving: 410 mg

Ingredients

☐ Spray of Grape-seed or Olive Oil

☐ Cipollini Onions (Peeled and Stemmed) 6

☐ Crimini Mushrooms (quartered)1 lb

☐ Water 4 quarts

☐ Whole Wheat or Gluten-free Fettuccine 6 ounces

☐ Low Sodium Chicken or Vegetable Broth ½ cup

☐ Salt ¼ tsp

☐ Fresh Ground Black Pepper

☐ Semi-soft Goat Cheese   1 ounce

☐ Porcini Dust 1 Tbsp

☐ Flat Leaf Parsley (Chopped)2 Tbsp

☐ Parmigiano-Reggiano (Grated)1 ounce

Directions

Preheat the oven to 375°F. Take two ovenproof pans and spray both of them with olive oil. In one pan put the onions and in the other put the mushrooms. Cover the pan with the onions and put both the pans into the preheated oven. Keep check on the mushrooms and keep stirring them after five minute intervals till they turn caramel in color. When the juices of the mushrooms evaporate, then they are nearly done.

In the meantime, boil the water in a stock pot and cook the fettuccine in it. Remove the mushrooms when they are done and add the stock, goat cheese, salt and pepper to the pan. Stir till the cheese melts. Then add the porcini dust over it and mix again.

Now take out the onions and put two onions in each serving bowl. Drain the cooked pasta and toss it with the mushrooms and sauce. If the sauce is too thick then dilute it with the pasta's cooking fluids. Drop in the parsley over the mixture. Now divide the pasta between the bowls that contain the onions and top off with grated Parmigiano-Reggiano.

Fettuccine with Roasted Red Pepper
Vinaigrette

Preparation Time: 10 minutes

Cooking Time: 30 minutes

Serving: 2 ounces pasta and 2/3 cup sauce serving for 4 people

Sodium per Serving: 499 mg

Ingredients

☐ Red Bell Peppers   3

☐ Spray Olive Oil

☐ White Onion (Diced)   1 large

☐ Garlic (Sliced) 2 cloves

☐ Dried rubbed Sage   2 tsp

☐ Curley Parsley (Coarsely chopped) ¼ cup

☐ Low Sodium Chicken or Vegetable Broth 1 cup

☐ Water ½ cup

☐ Salt ¼ tsp

☐ Fresh Ground Black Pepper (to taste)

☐ Balsamic Vinegar   2 tsp

☐ Extra Virgin Olive Oil   1 Tbsp

☐ Water 4 quarts

☐ Whole Wheat or Gluten-free Fettuccine 8 ounces

- [ ] Baby Arugula 2 cups
- [ ] Pecorino-Romano Cheese (grated) 2 ounces

Directions

Set the oven to broil and let it heat up. Roast the peppers in the oven and keep on turning it till the pepper is blackened all over. Remove it from the oven and place in a brown paper bag. Once it has cooled then peel it and deseed it. Then cut into strips.

Put the water in a large stock pot over high heat. Then heat up one tablespoon of olive oil in a large skillet over moderate flame. Stir fry the garlic and onions in it in it. When the onions have softened, then pour the stock and water over it. Add the red pepper, sage parsley, salt and pepper. Cook it for fifteen to twenty minutes, letting it simmer. Then remove it from heat and puree it with the help of a blender. Now return the smooth paste to the pan and pour in the olive oil and vinegar. Lower the heat to minimum.

Once the water has boiled up, put the fettuccine in. It should be cooked when it becomes tender. Once the fettuccine is done, drain it but reserve a quarter of a cup of the cooking liquid. Toss the fettuccine with the sauce and dilute it with the help of the reserved fluid.

Now increase the heat back to moderate and add the arugula to the saucepan. Cook with the new addition for one more minute and top with grated cheese when serving.

Fusilli with Morels and Roasted Garlic | Low Sodium Version

You need to make Roasted Garlic separately with this recipe. This recipe can be multiplied up to eight times but it can't be stored well.

Preparation Time: 10 minutes

Cooking Time: 20 minutes

Serving: 2 ounces serving for 2 people

Sodium per Serving: 386 mg

Ingredients

☐ Water 3 quarts

☐ Whole Wheat or Gluten-free Fusilli Pasta   4 ounces

☐ Olive Oil 1 Tbsp

☐ Shallot (Sliced lengthwise into thin strips)   1 large

☐ Fresh Morel Mushrooms8 ounces

☐ Roasted Garlic 8 ounces

☐ Salt 1/8 tsp

☐ Fresh Ground Black Pepper (to taste)

☐ Fresh Oregano 2 Tbsp

☐ Unsalted Butter 1 Tbsp

☐ Parmigiano-Reggiano (grated)1 ounce

Directions

Boil water in a large stock pot and put the fettuccine in. Let it cook.

While the pasta cooks, heat up one tablespoon of olive oil in a large skillet over moderate flame. Stir fry the olives in it. Then add the shallots and cook for three more minutes. Now add the already prepared roasted garlic to it and the mushrooms. Season with salt and pepper. Cook for five more minutes and toss frequently.

When the fusilli is don't, drain the pasta but reserve ½ cup of the cooking liquid. Add the pasta to the olive and mushrooms and throw in some oregano. Add the reserved liquid and mix up for a minute. Then add the butter. Let the butter melt before removing from heat.

Toss the pasta and serve it with a topping of shredded cheese.

Dessert

Creamy Peach Yogurt Pops

Yogurt pops can be a fun way of beating the heat and getting a nutritious healthy snack. Kids love them and adults can't resist either. The different flavors can be experimented with to suit the taste. This recipe can be doubled and tripled according to requirements.

Preparation Time: 10 minutes

Freezing Time: 3 hours

Serving: 1 ounce pop serving for 6 people

Sodium per Serving: 72 mg

Ingredients

☐ Fresh or Frozen Peaches 1 ½ cups

☐ Non-Fat Yogurt   2/3 cup

☐ 1% Cottage Cheese1/3 cup

☐ Granulated Stevia or Splenda ¼ cup

Directions

Blend together the yogurt, Splenda, peaches and cottage cheese. You should get a smooth puree in the end. If you do not have fresh peaches at hand

and are using frozen ones, then let them thaw for fifteen minutes before blending.

Now pour into freezer pop molds and either place a popsicle stick in each or the sticks that come with the molds. Freeze for around three hours to get solid pops.

In order to serve, run the molds upside down, under tap water and the pop will loosen and come out.

Grilled Pineapple with Creamy Balsamic Sauce

Pineapple has the ability to take you away to tropical paradise when you simply bite into it! So eat this treat when you want a break from every day routine. You can double or triple the recipe according to requirements and can store the leftover sauce for around two days.

Preparation Time: 10 minutes

Cooking Time: 20 minutes

Serving: 4 ounces serving for 2 people

Sodium per Serving: 24 mg

Ingredients

☐ Non-Fat Yogurt¼ cup

☐ Honey   1 Tbsp

☐ Pure Vanilla Extract ½ tsp

☐ Balsamic Vinegar 1 tsp

☐ Fresh Pineapple chunks 8 ounces

☐ Fresh Mint (finely chopped)

☐ Spray Grape-seed Oil

Directions

First of all blend together the yogurt, vanilla extract, vinegar and honey together with the help of a whisk. You can make this ahead of time and refrigerate it. Preheat the oven to 400°F and heat up a grill pan in it.

Arrange the pineapple chunks onto wooden skewers or cocktail sticks. Do not squash the chunks together but leave some gap between them.

When the pan has heated up, spray it lightly with the grape seed oil and place the skewers into the pan and sprinkle chopped mint over them. Pop the pan back into the oven and cook for fifteen minutes. Turn the skewers after every five minutes.

When serving, arrange the pineapple kebabs in small plates and drizzle the sauce over them or on the side.

Holiday Panna Cotta with Chocolate Cranberry Sauce

This dessert is meant for celebrations and holidays because it has a deep velvety taste that really gets you in the mood for enjoyment! You can triple the recipe if you are expecting guests and you can store the leftovers in the refrigerator for a couple of days.

Preparation Time: 20 minutes

Cooking Time: 20 minutes

Freezing Time: 4 hours

Serving: 1 panna cotta with sauce serving for 6 people

Sodium per Serving: 112 mg

Ingredients

☐ Warm Water2 Tbsp

☐ Unflavored Gelatin 1 ½ tsp

☐ 2% Milk 1 cup

☐ Sugar 2 Tbsp

☐ Honey 2 Tbsp

☐ Lemon Zest1 tsp

☐ Pure Vanilla Extract 2 tsp

☐ Ground Nutmeg 1 tsp

☐ Low-fat Buttermilk 2 cups

- ☐ Granulated Stevia or Splenda   2 Tbsp
- ☐ Sweetened dried Cranberries   ½ cup
- ☐ Water   2 cups
- ☐ Dark Chocolate1 ounce

Directions

Take two tablespoons of warm water and gently dust it with the gelatin. Do not mix it. In a non-reactive pan blend together the milk, sugar, vanilla extract, nutmeg, honey and lemon zest. Place it over moderate heat and bring it to a low boil. Reduce the heat and let it simmer for two minutes. Turn off the heat and as it cools take the gelatin and stir it into the milk. When the mixture is lukewarm, you can add the Splenda/stevia and the buttermilk to it.

Now take six ramekins and line them with cling film. Evenly divide the milk mixture between the prepared ramekins. Cover them individually and chill in the refrigerator for at least four hours.

While the panna cotta cools, you can cook the sauce. Take a non-reactive pan and pour water into it. Add the cranberries and bring it to a boil. Then lower the heat and allow it to simmer for an hour. There will be around a quarter cup of liquid left in the pan. Remove it from the heat and allow it to cool for ten minutes. Then pop in the entire bar of chocolate. After ten more minutes, the chocolate will be soft and gooey so that you can easily mix it up with the sauce.

When it is time to serve, take out the ramekins and invert them onto a serving plate. The dessert will easily come out and you can take off the plastic wrap. Serve with a helping of the cranberry chocolate sauce.

Homemade Fresh Caramel Popcorn

Whether it's the ball game or you are watching a movie, popcorn is necessary to add the entertainment. So why not indulge in a caramel coated treat the next time you are in front of the tube! The popcorn can be stored for a day but they are best when consumed fresh. Let the popcorn cool for fifteen minutes before tightly sealing them in plastic bags.

Cooking Time: 15 minutes

Serving: 5 cups serving for 3 people

Sodium per Serving: 233 mg

Ingredients

☐ Package Smart Balance Low Fat & Low Salt   1 Microwave Popcorn

☐ Caramel or Chocolate Ice Cream Topping   ¼ cup

Directions

You have to follow the instructions on the package of the microwavable popcorn for popping them. Usually it takes two and a half minutes on high power settings of the microwave.

Take a large mixing bowl and add the ice cream topping to it. The bowl should be large enough to hold the nearly fifteen cups of popcorn.

So once the popcorn is done, carefully open the bag to allow the steam to escape. Now heat the bowl with the topping for nearly a minute. But keep pausing the heating process after every ten seconds to ensure that the topping does not boil up or becomes too thin. Remove the bowl when the topping is warm and slowly moves when you tilt the bowl.

Now add the popcorn to the bowl and with the help if a rubber spatula, fold the popcorn with the sauce. Scrape the sides of the bowl and keep turning to coat all the popcorn with the sauce. Serve hot.

Key Lime Yogurt Pops

Yogurt pops can be a fun way of beating the heat and getting a nutritious healthy snack. Kids love them and adults can't resist either. The different flavors can be experimented with to suit the taste. This recipe can be doubled and tripled according to requirements.

Preparation Time: 10 minutes

Freezing Time: 3 hours

Serving: 1 pop serving for 4 people

Sodium per Serving: 81 mg

Ingredients

- ☐ Non-Fat Yogurt½ cup
- ☐ 1% Cottage Cheese ¼ cup
- ☐ Granulated Stevia or Splenda   ¼ cup
- ☐ Lime Juice¼ cup

Directions

Blend together the yogurt, Splenda, lime juice and cottage cheese. You should get a smooth puree in the end.

Now pour into freezer pop molds and either place a popsicle stick in each or the sticks that come with the molds. Freeze for around three hours to get solid pops.

In order to serve, run the molds upside down, under tap water and the pop will loosen and come out.

Peppermint Crème Brûlée

This is wonderful custard that can be served at formal gatherings and can be used as a delightful treat after dinner. It requires at least two days of preparation and cooking so if you wish to enjoy this custard, then you have to plan ahead. This recipe can be doubled and can be stored when wrapped tightly with cling film.

Cooking Time: 120 minutes

Serving: 1 custard serving for 4 people

Sodium per Serving: 199 mg

Ingredients

- ☐ 2% Milk 2 cups
- ☐ Non-Fat Dry Milk Powder½ cup
- ☐ Pure Vanilla Extract   1 tsp
- ☐ Fresh Peppermint Leaves8 large
- ☐ Granulated Splenda (or 7 Tbsp. Z-Sweet Stevia)   6 Tbsp
- ☐ Salt 1/8 tsp
- ☐ Egg Yolks 2 large
- ☐ Candy Canes 4 small

☐ Granulated Sugar   6 tsp

Directions

Use a non-reactive utensil or stainless steel pan for this recipe. Mix the dry milk powder and vanilla extract in the 2% milk. Heat the pan over moderate heat. Let the milk reach just boiling point and keep stirring to prevent it from boiling over. Now turn off the heat and add the peppermint leaves. Stir it a bit and let it cool for at least four hours in the refrigerator. Leaving them overnight is a good option.

Now preheat the oven to 300°F. You have to take a roasting pan and fill it with water, so that it will reach about ¾ the height of a one cup ramekin. You can place the ramekins in the pan and then fill it up to check the amount of water required. Once you have ensured the correct amount of water is in the pan, remove the ramekins from it and pop it in the preheated oven. Leave it in the oven for around twenty minutes to let it reach boiling point.

In a small stainless bowl, cream together the Splenda/Stevia, salt and egg yolks. Now take out the peppermint milk mixture from the refrigerator and sieve it through a fine sieve into the egg yolks. Throw away the mint leaves and whisk the yolks with the milk until you get a smooth paste.

Now evenly fill all four of the ramekins and take out the preheated water pan from the oven. Carefully place the ramekins into the pan and put the pan back into the oven. The cooking will take almost an hour.

Once the custard is done, very carefully ease out the pan and leave it to cool for half an hour, with the ramekins still in the water. Once cooled, take each ramekin and wrap it up with cling film. Let them chill in the refrigerator overnight.

Now powder the candy canes in a blender or chopper. Mix the sugar with two teaspoons of the candy cane powder. Now sprinkle two teaspoons of the sweet mixture over each chilled custard and melt it into crunch with the help of a blowtorch. Pay heed that the tip of the flame should be aimed at the points where the sugar is. You could pop the ramekins under the broiler to melt the sugar. But then you will have to allow the custard to cool on the counter for ten minutes and chill in the refrigerator for another twenty minutes.

Serve when the custard has cooled.

Strawberries with Balsamic Chocolate Sauce

Preparation Time: 10 minutes

Cooking Time: 40 minutes

Serving: ½ pint strawberries with 1 tablespoon sauce serving for 2 people

Sodium per Serving: 6 mg

Ingredients

☐ Balsamic Vinegar 1 cup

☐ Bittersweet Chocolate (Crumbled)2 ounces

☐ Pint Fresh Strawberries (rinsed, stemmed and sliced) 1

☐ Sugar 1 tsp

Directions

In order to reduce the balsamic vinegar, you will need a non-reactive saucepan or use a stainless steel utensil. Boil the vinegar over moderate heat and reduce the heat once the vinegar has reached boiling point. Let the vinegar simmer for around thirty to forty minutes to get ¼ cup. Let it cool slightly and then add the chocolate. Whisk it till the chocolate melts. Set it aside for half an hour.

During the reduction of the vinegar, combine the strawberries with the sugar to completely coat the slices. Leave it in the refrigerator for an hour.

When the strawberries are ready for serving, then fill up two bowls with the slices and top off with a teaspoon of the reduced balsamic chocolate sauce.

Strawberries with Balsamic Reduction

This recipe builds on the hint of sourness in the strawberries and presents an wonderful sauce. The balsamic vinegar reduced in this recipe is enough to be used for twelve individual servings. You can double the recipe or halve it.

Preparation Time: 10 minutes

Cooking Time: 40 minutes

Serving: ½ pint strawberries with 1 teaspoon sauce serving for 2 people

Sodium per Serving: 3 mg

Ingredients

☐ Balsamic Vinegar 1 cup

☐ Pint Fresh Strawberries (rinsed, stemmed and sliced) 1

☐ Sugar 1 tsp

☐ Fresh Ground Black Pepper

Directions

In order to reduce the balsamic vinegar, you will need a non-reactive saucepan or use a stainless steel utensil. Boil the vinegar over moderate heat and reduce the heat once the vinegar has reached boiling point. Let the vinegar simmer for around thirty to forty minutes to get ¼ cup. Let it cool.

During the reduction of the vinegar, combine the strawberries with the sugar to completely coat the slices. Leave it in the refrigerator for an hour.

When the strawberries are ready for serving, then fill up two bowls with the slices and top off with a teaspoon of the reduced balsamic vinegar and a dash of black pepper.

Strawberry Chocolate Sauce

Strawberries are a lovely sweet fruit with a hint of sourness. This lovely sauce can be used with desserts and cakes. You can triple the recipe and store the sauce in the refrigerator for up to three days.

Preparation Time: 10 minutes

Cooking Time: 20 minutes

Serving: ¼ cup serving for 4 people

Sodium per Serving: 1 mg

Ingredients

- ☐ Fresh Strawberries (Stemmed and Sliced)   4 ounces
- ☐ Water 1 cup
- ☐ Sugar 1 tsp
- ☐ Dutch Process Cocoa   2 Tbsp
- ☐ Semi-sweet Chocolate   ¾ ounce

Directions

First of all you will need a non-reactive utensil for cooking. Take any such saucepan and place the strawberries in it. Turn on medium heat under the pan and add water and sugar in it too. Simmer the strawberries for around twenty minutes.

When the strawberries are soft, remove from heat and let them cool. Puree with the help of a hand-held blender or a large blender. To ensure that no seeds or coarse parts stay in the sauce, pass it through a fine mesh sieve. Now put the sauce back in the pan and add the cocoa into the sauce. Blend it together and the melt the chocolate into the sauce. Remove from heat.

Place the sauce in the refrigerator for chilling at least an hour before serving.

Strawberry Sauce

Strawberries are a lovely sweet fruit with a hint of sourness. This lovely sauce can be used with desserts and cakes. You can triple the recipe and store the sauce in the refrigerator for up to three days.

Preparation Time: 10 minutes

Cooking Time: 20 minutes

Serving: ¼ cup serving for 4 people

Sodium per Serving: 0 mg

Ingredients

☐ Fresh Strawberries (Stemmed and Sliced)   4 ounces

☐ Water 1 cup

☐ Sugar 1 tsp

Directions

First of all you will need a non-reactive utensil for cooking. Take any such saucepan and place the strawberries in it. Turn on medium heat under the pan and add water and sugar in it too. Simmer the strawberries for around twenty minutes.

When the strawberries are soft, remove from heat and let them cool. Puree with the help of a hand-held blender or a large blender. To ensure that no seeds or coarse parts stay in the sauce, pass it through a fine mesh sieve. Place the sauce in the

refrigerator for chilling at least an hour before
serving.

Hearts Parmesan Salad

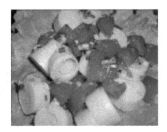

INGREDIENTS

- 1 (14 ounce) cans hearts of palm, drained & rinsed
- 2 medium tomatoes, seeded & chopped
- 3 garlic cloves, finely chopped
- 2 green onions, chopped (use white & green parts)
- 2 tablespoons extra virgin olive oil
- Salt and pepper (Use fresh cracked pepper)
- 2 ounces parmesan cheese, freshly shaved
- 2 tablespoons fresh basil, chopped

DIRECTIONS

- First of all cut the center of foist into 2/3 wide slice combine all but the parmesan and together ingredients in a large bowl throw and let to sit at room temperature for about 28 minutes let the taste to cuter treat with shavings of parmesan on best of the salad.

Heart Healthy Bean Pasta

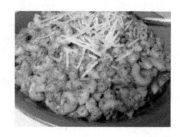

INGREDIENTS

- 1 lb cavatappi pasta, cooked according to directions
- 1/2 cup lima beans, defrosted
- 2 -3 garlic cloves
- 1 1/2 cups fresh basil, packed
- 1/2 cup baby arugula, packed
- 1 cup parmesan-Romano cheese mix, grated
- 1/4 cup part-skim ricotta cheese
- 1/2 cup olive oil
- Sriracha hot chili sauce (optional)

DIRECTIONS

- First of all into a hurry blender set lima beans and garlic stir arugula basil and butter pulsate to cuter slow stir oil about food tube to make a nice beat harden with nutrition and sriracha pepper to your heat even throw into warm browned cavatappi pasta spot with scrape butter and see it vanish.

Peppermint Latte Heart Healthy

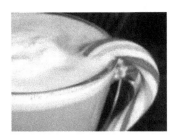

INGREDIENTS

- 1 cup nonfat milk
- 1 tablespoon creme de menthe coffee syrup or 1 tablespoon peppermint schnapps or 1 tablespoon crème de menthe
- 1/2 cup espresso coffee (prepared)
- Sugar (optional) or Splendid sugar substitute (optional)
- 2 tablespoons frozen light whipped dessert topping, thawed (such as light Cool Whip)
- 2 peppermint stick candy

DIRECTIONS

- First of all in a normal pepper pan heat and add the milk till warm but not abscess add in the crème de menthe syrup or peppermint schnapps hurry to make frothy divide espresso between 3 large cups divide milk between the 3 cups if true specify with sugar or splendid best several servings with whipped best and add with a peppermint thrust treat away.

Heart and Tomato Salad

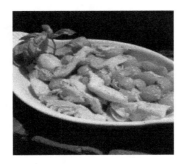

INGREDIENTS

- 4 ripe medium tomatoes
- 8 canned artichoke hearts (not marinated)
- 1/4 cup olive oil
- 1 tablespoon wine vinegar
- 1 garlic clove, pressed (optional)
- 1 tablespoon fresh tarragon (or a 1/4 tsp dried)
- 1 tablespoon fresh basil (or 1/4 tsp dried)
- 2 tablespoons feta cheese
- Salt
- Pepper

DIRECTIONS

- First of all cut each tomato into 5 wedges and each artichoke into halves cuter the base of the ingredients and together pour slice the vegetables toss refrigerate for about 18 minutes.

185

Mushrooms and Artichoke Hearts Vinaigrette

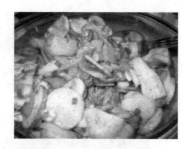

INGREDIENTS

- 2 (6 ounce) jars marinated artichoke hearts
- 2 (7 1/2 ounce) cans sliced water chestnuts, drained
- 1 lb fresh mushrooms, thinly sliced
- 1 bunch scallion, chopped
- 2 tablespoons olive oil
- 1 1/2 tablespoons balsamic vinegar
- 1/2 teaspoon salt
- 1 dash black pepper
- 1 dash hot pepper sauce

DIRECTIONS

- First of all tire artichokes keep the marinade from shake place the artichokes in a normal bowl stir water chestnuts mushrooms and together scallions stir olive oil vinegar nutrition and warm pepper to silent artichoke marinade hurry easily to cuter pour slices vegetables and throw treat away or coat and marinate in chill for up to 2 days enjoy.

Hearts of Palm Guacamole

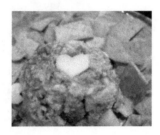

INGREDIENTS

- 1 (14 ounce) cans hearts of palm, drained
- 1/2-3/4 cup cilantro, packed
- 2 -3 fresh garlic cloves, minced
- 1/2 lemon, juice of
- 1 tablespoon olive oil
- 3 avocados
- 1 teaspoon ground cumin, more to taste
- 1/4 teaspoon salt, more to taste
- 1/2 teaspoon ground black pepper, more to taste
- 1/2 cup red onion, chopped (optional)
- 1/2 cup tomatoes, chopped (optional)
- Jalapenos (if heat is desired) or cayenne pepper, to taste (if heat is desired)

DIRECTIONS

- First of all place hearts of fist cilantro chop garlic lemon juice and olive oil in a normal bowl use an immersion food processor to puree juicer could be used also clutter the avocados into the puree combine with the back of a spend add in fragrance add in tomato and onion and jalapeno or cayenne if true use it just as you would orderly guacamole.

Buenos Hearts Salad

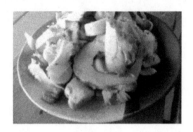

INGREDIENTS

- 1 (14 ounce) cans hearts of palm, thinly sliced
- 1 tomatoes, thinly sliced
- 1 avocado, quartered and thinly sliced
- 1/4 cup extra virgin olive oil
- 1 tablespoon fresh orange juice
- 1 tablespoon fresh lime juice
- Salt and pepper

DIRECTIONS

- First of all on a platter order the hearts of foist tomato and avocado in a single outer slosh layer in a small bowl whip together the olive oil orange juice and lime juice harden with nutrition and sauce sprinkle the bandage outer the salad.

Healthy Heart Muffins

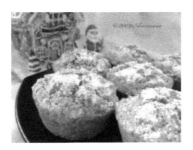

INGREDIENTS

- 3 egg whites
- 3/4 cup skim milk
- 1 cup low-fat yogurt
- 3/4 cup applesauce
- 2 cups whole meal flour
- 1/2 cup rolled oats
- 1/2 cup oat bran
- 3 teaspoons baking powder
- 2 teaspoons cinnamon
- 3/4 cup raisins
- 3/4 cup dried apricot, diced

DIRECTIONS

- First of all stir liquid to dry ingredients and together combine with care spoon into muffin tins spoon into muffin tins preheat 175 C for about 21 minutes hammer egg palliate easily stir milk yoghurt and apple pepper.

CPSIA information can be obtained
at www.ICGtesting.com
Printed in the USA
LVHW080300291122
734234LV00035B/1838